Md. Matiur Rahman
Md. Aminur Rahman
Md. Rahidul Islam

Responses of the Community People towards COVID-19: A Rapid Assessment

Md. Matiur Rahman
Md. Aminur Rahman
Md. Rahidul Islam

Responses of the Community People towards COVID-19: A Rapid Assessment

LAP LAMBERT Academic Publishing

Publisher:
LAP LAMBERT Academic Publishing
is a trademark of
International Book Market Service Ltd., member of OmniScriptum Publishing Group
17 Meldrum Street, Beau Bassin 71504, Mauritius
Printed at: see last page
ISBN: 978-620-2-81576-5

ACKNOWLEDGEMENT

First and foremost, we would like to extend our heartiest thanks and gratitude to **Professor Dr. Hosne-Ara Begum**, Ashoka Fellow & AKS, the Founder Executive Director of TMSS for her continuous support and inspirations. Words of appreciation are extended to **Professor Dr. Moudud Hossain Alamgir**, Executive Advisor, Research Planning and Development, TMSS Health Sector for encouraging us to initiate this study.

Additionally, we would like to extend our sincere appreciation to all the study respondents from the various communities for providing their willful contributions through providing valuable information on COVID19 issues with very patience. All the research assistants and data enumerators who conducted the interviews of the respondents in the field are highly acknowledged with gratitude. We would like to acknowledge the contributions of Mr. Md. Nahid Hossen, Assistant Director and Coordinator, TMSS Health Care Center (THCC) and his Departments for extensive cooperation and continuous support in implementing data collection and sincere commitment towards fulfilling this research endeavor. Besides, no thanks are sufficient for TMSS HEM Sector, without whose support this assessment could not be completed.

We would like to acknowledge the support of the MIS & Documentation Department of TMSS Health Sector on different issues. The authors are also gratefully acknowledging the sincere support of Health Sector Secretariat, and Finance and Account of TMSS Health Sector.

ACRONYMS

CBO	Community-based Organization
HHs	House Holds
NGO	Non-governmental Organization
RP&D	Research, Planning & Development
THCC	TMSS Health Care Center
THS	TMSS Health Sector
TMSS	Thengamara Mohila Sabuj Sangha
WHO	World Health Organization

EXECUTIVE SUMMARY

This study has been conducted on a special significance on health issues that is COVID-19 Pandemic, very important at present. During COVID-19 Pandemic, TMSS HEALTH SECTOR (THS) has organized a study with several challenges entitled, RESPONSES OF THE COMMUNITY PEOPLE TOWARDS COVID-19: A RAPID ASSESSMENT. When Bangladesh is crippling with COVID-19 and meanwhile more than two thousand (since study) people have been died and spread diseases all over the country including rural and urban both. Out of Dhaka, Bogura is one district town and sub-urban areas where COVID-19 disease has been spread over and thousands of people have been infected with the Coronavirus and for this, TMSS authority has converted its Medical College Hospital[1] as COVID HOSPITAL immediately for providing the services to the COVID-19 patients. When the whole social environment is fearful then THS has taken also a decision to conduct a study on COVID-19 pandemic in order to understand deeply why people have been infected massively by Corona Virus that helps also for taking steps both preventive and curative as a treatment procedure. The basic concentration of this Rapid Assessment is 'to search the knowledge level on COVID-19, to examine the practices of the local people in protecting Coronavirus, to know the types of problem people have been faced during lock-down and know the suggestions of the study population on policies and procedural actions'.

In conducting the study, a total of 639 respondents (Male-259/40.5% & Female-380/59.8%) have been interviewed through semi-structured questionnaires with random sampling. Considering the limitation of the lock-down situation, face to face interview has been conducted, that was a crucial challenge for this study, but overcome the challenges with mitigating the loopholes. In the educational attainment of the respondents, only 9.7% are illiterate where primary passed 26.8%, JSC 21.4%, and SSC 17.7%. Regarding this, 10.5% respondents have HSC passed and 9.4% have the Honors degree also. The similar scenario is seen on occupational status where 46.3% women respondents are housewives who have no direct income, but 21.4% are service holders and 11.9% are businessmen. In considering the importance, 5 Health Professionals (Physician, Nurse, other Health Workers) have contributed to this study though the percentage is very poor, only .8% and student's contributions are 5.2%.

Respondent's Knowledge about Corona Virus is one of the prime objectives of this study; and according to the information, it has seen that 88.9% have claimed, they know about the Coronavirus that represents 568 respondents in frequency. Three

---

[1] It is known also as Rafatullah Community Hospital

matters have been considered in this regard that includes 'transmission process of Coronavirus, knowledge about major symptoms of the COVID-19 and after how many days it will appear'. Regarding transmission, most of the respondents (34.3%) have claimed, 'by contact with contaminated surfaces (sneeze, cough, phlegm, cold, etc. of infected persons) and 25.1% informed, 'talking closely with infected persons' where 21.6% claimed that 'through the Air'. 13.1% respondents have informed Coronavirus has been transmitted person to person due to 'lack of hygiene care of infected people' and 2.1% thought, 'through sexual contact'. On knowledge about symptoms of Coronavirus, 92.0% have claimed. 'they know the symptoms'. As their opinion, major symptoms are 'Fever (29.7%), Shortness of breathing (23.7%), Sore throat (16.8%) and Cough (13.6%). When they are asked, after how many days these symptoms are appeared, 87.5% respondents said, 'after 8-14 days' and 12.5% informed, 'during 1-7 days'.

Regarding Corona infected Family Members and Neighbors, only 54 respondents (8.5%) have informed, their family members have been infected with Coronavirus. And it is seen, 11 respondents infected with Corona (20.4%), and Spouse and Parents both numbers are 8 (14.8%) who are infected also. In addition, 11.1% 'Brother and Sister (6) and 2 children also infected. Through this information, it has revealed that all types of kins are infected though the figure is not high. In this category, 'other relatives' has occupied a major number that is 35.2% (19) among total infected 54. When it has been searched how many neighbors have been infected with Corona, 11.9% (76) claimed, their neighbors are infected with Coronavirus. Death number is very important to know the comparative ratio to the infected patients; according to the data, 13 have been lost their lives though infected was 54.

One of the major objectives of this Rapid Assessment has tried to know preventive measures that have been taken to protect COVID-19. And it has seen 40.1% practiced 'hand washing or using hand sanitizer last three days of survey date' sometimes,

When they have been asked, whether they have access to sources in getting COVID-19 information, 54% have said full access and 42.6% informed 'partially access'; but 3.4% have said 'they have no access in any sources in knowing information on COVID-19. Additionally, they have identified key sources like 'electronic and print media; where 78.9% have access, 60.6% access to NGO Workers, 44% access to neighbors, relatives and friends and 40% claimed to Health Workers. Out of this, they have taken information through 'leaflet/miking (24.7%), social media (22.5%) and religious leaders (10.6%)'. The important issue is, 63.1% have claimed they have knowledge for preventing COVID-19 whereas 40% did not have the knowledge. How possible to enhance the knowledge of the study population, mostly (44.4%) suggested. 'courtyard meeting can be organized', 28.8% said for 'miking could be increased', and 6.8% advocated for 'to increase distribution of poster/leaflet and flyers.

Regarding the impact of COVID-19 on people's income and livelihood is another important area to search with how and which extent. Most of the respondents (94.2%) has been suffered with bad impact on earning that hampers their access to food and other daily facilities. When this study wanted to know the frequency of reducing their income, it has known, salary has been decreased between before and during COVID period as like before COVID-21.9% & COVID period -14.9%, in agro-sector, during COVID, 31.8% respondents claimed decreased and the same decreasing scenario has been identified for Daily laborers the figure are before COVID -19.1% and during COVID-15.%. The earning scenario has been decreased under COVID-19 lock-down and peoples' sufferings have been downtrodden immensely. Now try to know how they have cope-up with, according to assessment, 4.1% informed, 'through assistance of family, relatives and friends and 7.4% informed through the social safety net. But 3.9% respondents informed, they have passed their days during COVID-19, without having any income.

Regarding monthly income whose earning was from 10,000 BDT to 50,000 BDT, it has been decreased approximately. When respondents informed about experiencing problems it is seen 7% claimed, lost their jobs, 29.1% 'closed their shop', 22.7% 'lost their livelihood capital' but 88.7% claimed, 'experienced income drop'. Now the question is how they have coped up with when income has been dropped seriously. As assessment, mostly 'borrowed from relatives/neighbors/friends, loan from informal institutions and CBOs and some of them sold jewelry or valuable assets. But 61.3% said, 'they have lessened their meals for coping the decreased income.

For any pandemic, access to healthcare is very important and it has seen that 67.6% respondents have faced health problem during COVID-19 that includes 'physical illness, severe stress and mental illness mostly. Regarding getting healthcare, data indicates a negative analysis of access to health institutions. Accessibility ratio has been lessened as '-35.29/community clinic, -38.40/government hospital, -42.30/private hospitals and -28.42 lost access to the mobile clinic. It indicates, respondents have lost their right to access to health institutions in getting healthcare facilities. What are the reasons that responsible for not access to Health Institutions during COVID-19 pandemic, three major reasons have been identified; those are 'unavailable transport to reach health institutions (41.7%), did not go to health institutes for fear of infection by Coronavirus (30.3%) and Doctors are not available (11.1%)'.

During COVID-19 pandemic, Mother and children have been suffered immensely in taking health services, according to the Rapid Assessment, 70.6% informed, they failed to get health services from any health institutes. Reasons behind that 'unavailable transport to reach health institutions (30.8%), did not go to health institutes for fear of infection by Coronavirus (37.4%) and Health institutes are open but refrained from providing any service (12.7%). That means mothers and children have been failed to get any services due to the COVID-19 pandemic.

On Humanitarian Assistance, for mitigating people's basic needs and crises, government and many non-government organizations have allocated several types of assistance for those who have needed supports. As information, among 639 respondents 24.9% (159) have claimed they got assistance during the COVID-19 period and 67.4% claimed, 'they got 'dry rations like rice, potato, oil and vegetable', 11.5% informed, 'money includes hand cash and Cheque and near about 10% informed, 'hygiene packs like Sanitizer, Savlon, Mask, etc. The authority who provided assistance as like government (41.2%), NGOs (39.2%), Local clubs/Institutions/Societies (16.7%), and from rich man 02.9%.

Finally, through the whole analysis, many crises and hopes have been revealed that people have experienced during the COVID-19 pandemic. But the respondents have also suggested what should be done during pandemic like COVID-19. Based on the respondent's suggestions, Researcher's observation, few recommendations are presented here as follows:

- Awareness programs should be introduced among the people on COVID-19 and its impact.
- COVID-19 test opportunities should be practiced in rural areas especially among poor people.
- Assistance and the safety-net program should be expanded during any pandemic.
- Treatment of corona-infected poor people should be lessened or freed.
- Alternative livelihood approach should be introduced when lockdown is imposed.
- Health Care Institutes could be opened all time during any pandemic.
- Health Card may be introduced for the marginal people as like the safety-net program.
- People should be involved personally and the community as a whole to take further steps to remove the stigma and do practices health safety rules in the COVID perspective.

CONTENTS

LIST OF TABLES

LIST OF FIGURES

Introduction

CHAPTER ONE

CHAPTER ONE
INTRODUCTION

1.1 INTRODUCTION

With the outbreak of novel coronavirus-2 (nCoV-2) declared a global pandemic and an international public health emergency by the World Health Organization (WHO). The entire world is working to address it. It is a rapidly evolving and emerging situation. In 5 months after the first emergence of the virus in December 2019, more than seven million people in 213 countries and territories around the globe have been identified as confirmed cases of coronavirus (COVID-19) where almost 3.61 million people have recovered and more than 0.4 million deaths have been reported (Worldometers, 2020). Researchers across the world are working hard to understand better the biology of nCoV-2 and the epidemiology of the novel coronavirus disease-19 (COVID-19). The estimated basic reproductive number of the virus is significantly higher than many other infectious diseases, and this can potentially result in the capacity of health facilities becoming overwhelmed, even in the countries that have the most developed healthcare systems (Li Q, 2020). An estimated 20% of cases lead to clinically serious and complex conditions. With some sporadic cases of serious illness in younger individuals, adults >60 years of age and with co-morbid conditions make up the most vulnerable group.

There are as yet no vaccines or specific antiviral drugs approved for the disease, and hence, nontherapeutic interventions to control the spread of the virus are the most effective measures to control the disease (Bootsma MCJ, Ferguson NM, 2007). Worldwide, billions of people are staying at home to minimize the transmission of the virus. Many countries are adopting preventive measures, e.g., remote office activities, international travel bans, mandatory lockdowns, and social distancing. Bangladesh, a middle-income country and one of the world's most densely populated areas, is struggling to combat the spread of the disease.

COVID-19 pandemic was confirmed to have started spreading in Bangladesh since March 2020 (IEDCR, 2020). Since then the new infections grew exponentially and now the rate is highest in Asia along with wider community-level transmission. To stop the spread of this virus, there are lots of actions taken by the government like quarantine throughout the local and countrywide, travel restriction, Hazard control in the workplace, cancellation and postponements of events, border enclosure and screening at airports, etc. These kinds of preventive measures like lockdown may hinder the normal flow of raw materials, products, and services, capitals, humans which resulting in business and production shutdowns at least temporarily (Barua, 2020). This pandemic has led to acute global socioeconomic disruption such as extensive fear of supply shortage resulting in panic buying. To prevent the outbreak of coronavirus, the Government of Bangladesh also declared 10 days general holiday firstly on 22 March which is effective from 26 March later the holiday has been extended 5 more times to 30 May 2020. As of July 31, 2020, the Government of Bangladesh has confirmed testing 1176809 samples among which there are a total of 237661 confirmed cases, nearly 135136 recoveries, and more than 3 thousand deaths in the country (IEDCR, 2020). In Bangladesh, the preventive measures have been found challenging to implement due to a lack of general awareness of COVID-19 and the absence of a social safety net.

In Bogura, a district city of northern Bangladesh is now under threatening of COVID-19 pandemic and meanwhile, many citizens have been detected as corona virus infected. Besides, due to the COVID-19 pandemic, people have faced rare experiences where their normal livelihood is halted. Evidence shows that 'earnings, transportation, treatment, movement, farming, business and other IGAs have been postponed for declared strict lockdown and quarantine since March 2020. And peoples' sufferings are beyond imagination and it may predict both urban and rural people have been under misery situation that collapses their basic needs, fully and partially. Considering the human-disaster, the Research Department of TMSS Health Sector has taken a rapid study entitled, 'Responses of the Community people towards COVID-19: A Rapid Assessment' to know the impact of COVID-19 on peoples' lives who is living in Bogura and adjacent districts town and sub-urban and rural areas.

1.2 OBJECTIVES OF THE STUDY

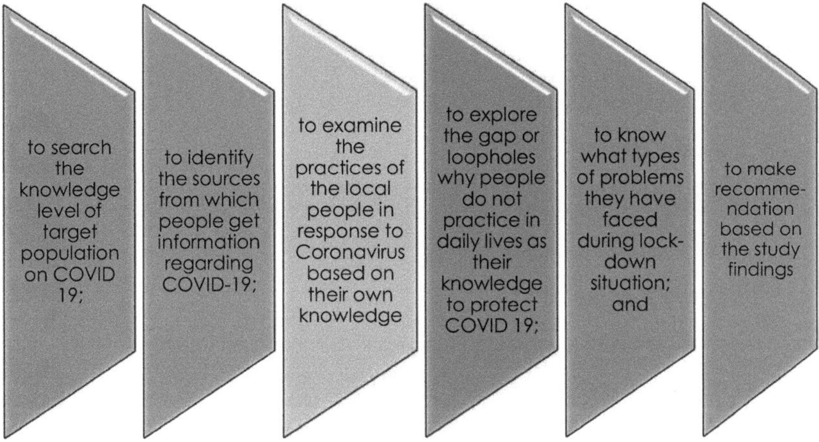

1.3 RATIONALE OF THE STUDY

This study helps to assess the knowledge and attitudes of people towards the Covid-19 disease. This study helps to find out the knowledge gaps among the people regarding the Covid-19 and the misconceptions and superstitious beliefs prevailing in the society about it.

This study also provides descriptive data that may be useful for the concerned authority and planning institutions while preparing plans and programs to tackle the Covid-19 disease. Also, after this study people will be aware of adopting healthy lifestyles and can manage and prevent complications.

1.4 LIMITATIONS OF THE STUDY

- The time of data collection was very short making it difficult to undertake detailed responses against all issues.
- The study did not include respondents from the whole northern part of Bangladesh except Bogura, Naogaon, Gaibandha, and Joypurhat Districts.
- Due to lockdown, data collection was extremely challenging.

METHODS AND MATERIALS

Introduction

Study Design

Study Places

Study Period

Study population

Sample Size Determination and Distribution

Sources of Data

Procedure of Data Collection

Data Management

Data Analysis Techniques

Ethical Issues

CHAPTER TWO

CHAPTER TWO
METHODS AND MATERIALS

2.1   INTRODUCTION

This chapter briefly describes the methodology that is used in the present study. It includes research approach and design, description of the study place along with the sampling techniques, sample size and sampling frame, data collection procedure, tools and techniques, and all other related issues to the study. Besides, data editing, coding, data analysis, and ethical consideration of the study have also been provided in this chapter.

2.2   STUDY DESIGN

The study is a community based cross-sectional design. Quantitative technique has been used to collect information from respective respondents. And a semi-structured questionnaire has been used for collecting the necessary data and information from the targeted respondents.

2.3   STUDY PLACES

The study has been carried out in the four (4) Districts of Rajshahi and Rangpur Divisions namely Bogura, Gaibandha, Joypurhat, and Naogaon. All these four Districts have been chosen purposively because the majority of the TMSS Health Care Centers (64 out of 86) are operated in these areas.

2.4   STUDY PERIOD

The study has been conducted for a period of 3 months (June 2020 to August 2020). First Month (June) has been used for Protocol and Tools Development. Data Collection, Coding, and Analysis have been performed in the second month of study, and the last month has been used to prepare the draft report and the final report has also been submitted after internal and external review in the same month.

2.5   STUDY POPULATION

Before selecting a sample size, researcher has to demarcate a population. For meeting the study objectives, the people of community (men and women with more than 18 years old) who are the beneficiaries of TMSS Health Care Center have been taken as the population of the study for data and information collection.

2.6   SAMPLE SIZE DETERMINATION AND DISTRIBUTION

To achieve the objectives of the study, multistage sampling techniques have been applied. At first, four (4) catchment Districts of the TMSS Health Care Center (THCC) have been taken purposively which is Bogura, Joypurhat, Naogaon, and Gaibandha. One-fourth of the total branches of THCC operated in the above-mentioned area have been taken randomly for this study and which are 16 branches (out of 64bBranches). These 16 branches have been distributed vided proportionately among the four Districts (in Bogura 10 out of 41, In Gaibandha 3 out of 11, in Joypurhat 2 out of 10, and Naogaon 1 out of 2 Branches). After that, equal number of respondents have been interviewed from each THCC following the same methods.

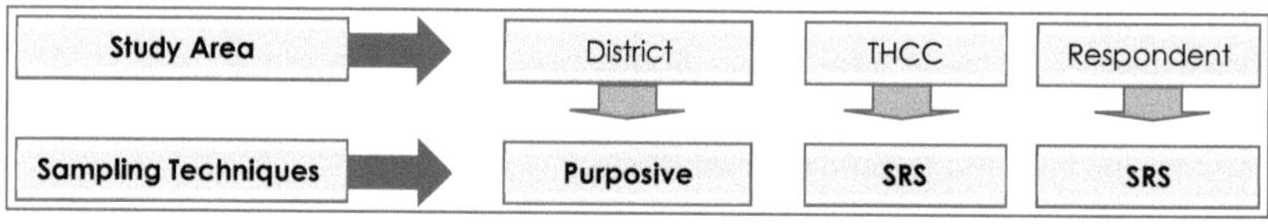

Figure 2. 1: Study Area Selection Process

The sample size has been calculated by applying the single population proportion formula, using a proportion of 0.5 and expected margin of error=0.05, based on the following formula-

The formula is:

n   = z2pq/d2

       = (1.96)2×.50×.50/0.052

       = 384

Where;

n= Desired sample size (if the target population is less than 10,000);

z= The standard normal deviation at the required confidence level (in this case 1.96 and which is 95% confidence level);

p= Estimated population proportion. To get the maximum sample size p was taken as 50% (P=0.5);

q= 1-p; and

d= The level of statistical significance set

Therefore, the calculated sample size is 384. But in this study, 639 respondents have been interviewed as sample for better and more accurate result and the distribution has been provided as below-

Table 2.1: Sample Branches of TMSS Health Care Centers (THCC)

SL. No	Name of THCC Branches	No of Respondents
01	Gokul	40
02	Matidali	40
03	Ashekpur	40
04	Sherpur	40
05	Velurpara	40
06	Sonamuya	39
07	Zianagor	40
08	Jaypurhut	40
09	Punat	40
10	Sherrotty	40
11	Molamgari	40
12	Jamalgonj	40
13	Komorpur	40
14	Mohimagonj	40
15	Barokona	40
16	Nawgaon	40
Total	**16 THCC Branches**	**639**

2.7 SOURCES OF DATA

Primary data has been used in this study. Data has been collected from the respondents in the proposed study area using questionnaire survey.

2.8 PROCEDURE OF DATA COLLECTION

2.8.1 Questionnaire Survey

A semi-structured questionnaire has been developed after pre-testing having both close-ended and open-ended questions which have been used to collect relevant data. The questionnaire has been divided into seven parts including participant socio-demographic information, knowledge of COVID-19, practice regarding COVID-19, the impact of lockdown, etc. Sufficient time has been given to respondents to read, comprehend, and answer all the questions. A group of trained research assistants has been approached the respondents, ask question and write down the answers in front of respondents.

2.9 DATA MANAGEMENT

Only relevant, accurate, unbiased representative data has been gathered from reliable sources. The data collected through the field survey has been compiled, tabulated, and coded to tailor to the objectives of the study. Data has been analyzed and interpreted using appropriate statistical methods with modern application software IBM SPSS 25 Version.

2.10 DATA ANALYSIS TECHNIQUES

2.10.1 Statistical Tools

A descriptive statistical method has been used in this study for analyzing data. The descriptive analyses include frequency distribution, mean, maximum, minimum, etc. have been used in this study.

2.10.2 Graphical Representation

Graphical representation of a frequency is more effective than tabular representation & it is also easily understandable. Diagram is essential to convey the statistical information to the general public. It is also facilitating the comparison of two or more frequency distribution. It considers some important types of graphical representation, such as bar diagrams, pie charts, etc.

2.11 ETHICAL CONSIDERATION

Ethical issues are an important part of research. The research team has strictly maintained all the ethical issues which are related to research in every stage of the study. Before collecting data, respondents were informed about the objectives of research and their prior permission and privacy were ensured. On the other hand, it was assured to the respondents that this information will only be used for academic research purpose and their name and designation will never be used for any other purpose.

The Page is intentionally left blank

RESULT AND ANALYSIS

Socio-economic and Demographic Information of Respondent

Family Related Information of the Respondents

Respondent'S Knowledge about Novel Coronavirus

Infection of Coronavirus among the Family Members and Neighbor

Preventive Measures Practiced by the Respondent

Sources of COVID-19 Related Information

Impact of COVID-19 on Livelihood, Income and Food In-take

Impact on Accessibility of Essential Health Care Services

Access to Aid/Distribution of Humanitarian Assistance

CHAPTER THREE

CHAPTER THREE
RESULT AND ANALYSIS

SECTION-1: SOCIO-ECONOMIC AND DEMOGRAPHIC INFORMATION OF THE RESPONDENTS

For any study, respondent's basic information is very important to understand the livelihood situation in which they belong. This Rapid Assessment has contained the information considering sex, age, religion, education, marriage, occupation and living areas also. Here it describes all the issues in detail.

Figure 3.1.1: Distribution of the Respondents by the Sex

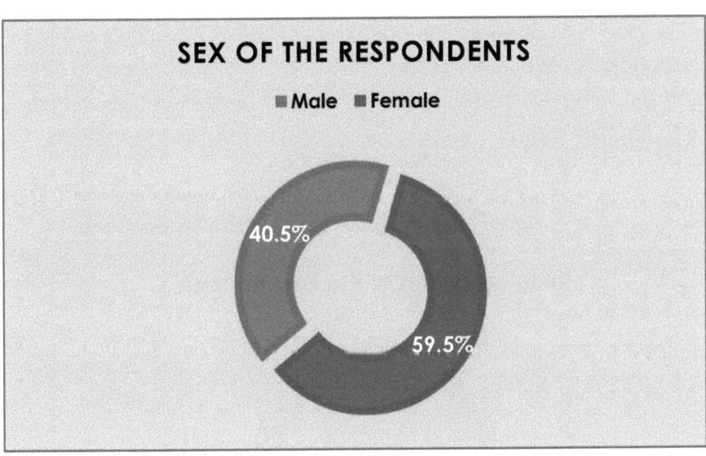

The given figure 3.3.1 illustrates the distribution of the respondents based on their biological construction, popularly called sexual identification. The total number of respondents is 639 where 59.5 percent of the respondents is women, and 40.5 percent of respondents is men. And it is observed that female respondents are higher than male respondents among total respondents.

Age is another variable that helps us to understand the nature and difference of the respondents and it links to knowledge and practices also, as human being. Figure 3.1.2 shows the distribution of the respondents in respect to their age group in years with frequencies and percentages. It also illustrates that there is a total of 639 respondents and among them, 37.7% belongs to the age group of 21-30 years and 34.9% belongs to the age group 31-40 years.

Figure 3.1.2: Distribution of the Respondents by their age

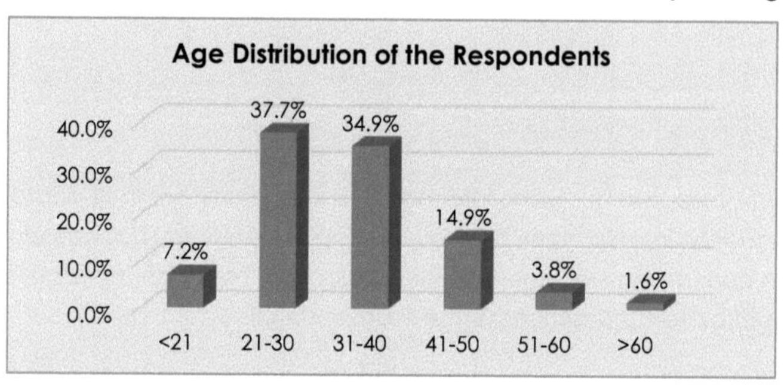

It is seen that only 1.6 percent of the respondents is above 60 years, and 3.8 percent is from the age of 51-60 years. The age group of below 21 years and 41-50 years of the respondents are 7.2 percent and 14.9 percent respectively. Majority percentage of the respondents among the total number of respondents is youth according to their age.

Figure 3.1.3: Religious Status of the Respondents

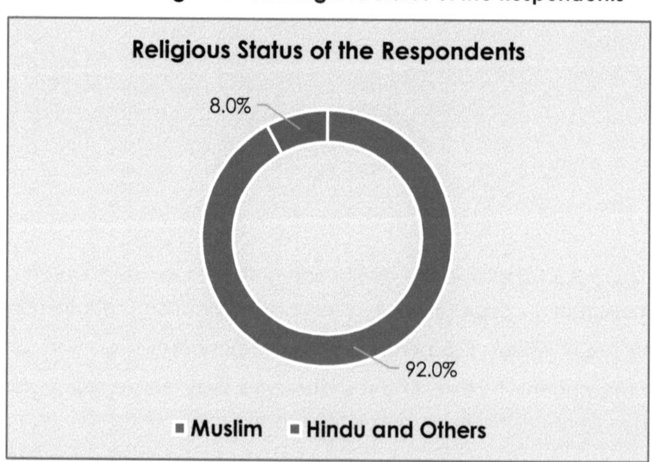

Regarding religious status of the respondents, figure 3.1.3 states that among 639 respondents, 92% respondents are Muslim and 8 percent are Hindu and others. In terms of religion point of view of the respondents, Muslim is big numbers rather than Hindu and other religions.

Educational qualification is another variable that has been used to know the people's psychological construction, survival strategy and social status, as well.

Table 3.1.1: Educational Qualification of the Respondents

Educational Status	n	%
Illiterate	62	9.7
Primary	171	26.8
JSC	137	21.4
SSC	113	17.7
HSC	67	10.5
Honors	60	9.4
Masters	28	4.4
Others	1	0.2
Total	639	100

According to the table 3.1.1, it is seen level of education of the respondents where 26.8 percent who have completed their primary education. On the other hand, it has revealed, 21.4 percent, 17.7 percent, and 10.5 percent respondents have completed JSC, SSC and HSC respectively. Besides, only 4.4% respondents have passed Master Degree where 0.2% achieved masters-above, while the number of the respondents who has completed their bachelor degree is 9.4 percent. But it has known, 9.7% respondents are illiterate.

On marital status, table 3.1.2 states that 89.8% respondents are married where divorced and separated are 0.5 percent in each among total 639 respondents.

Table 3.1.2: Marital Status of the Respondents

Marital Status	n	%
Single	48	7.5
Married	574	89.8
Divorced	3	0.5
Widowed	11	1.7
Separated	3	0.5
Total	639	100

It has known also that 7.5 percent respondents are single and 1.7 percent respondents are separated also. It is clearly seen that majority percent of the respondents are married in this regard.

For any study, respondent's occupation is very important for analyzing their living standard and social status that they belong during study.

Table 3.1.3: Occupational Status of the Respondents

Occupation	n	%
Service Holder	137	21.4
Health Professional	5	0.8
Business	76	11.9
Farming	43	6.7
Day Labor	20	3.1
Unemployed	15	2.3
House Wife	296	46.3
Student	33	5.2
Others	14	2.2
Total	**639**	**100**

Table 3.1.3 illustrates the occupational status of the respondents and 46.3% have been identified as house wives (n=296) and 21.4% are service holders (n=137). 'Unemployment' is identified here as 2nd lowest out of 639 respondents that represents 2.3% while 'other categories' occupied 2.2% percent, the lowest. Rest of the occupations namely day labor, student, farming, physician workers, and business are 3.1%, 5.2%, 6.7%, 8% and 11.9% respectively.

For the nature of the study, living areas of the respondents is considered important also in here. According to figure 3.1.4, most of the respondents have been living in rural areas that is 78.1 percent but 6.1 percent respondents are living in Upazila town.

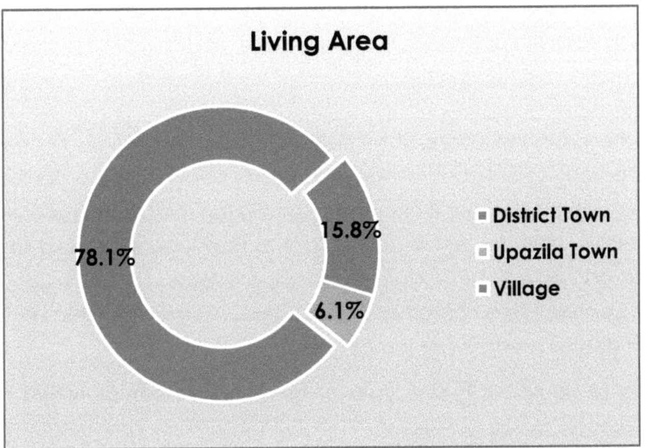

Regarding urban area, 15.8 percent have been living in District town where 6.1 percent at Upazila town. But 78.1 percent respondents are living at Village. It indicates that the findings of this study have been portrayed a mixed scenario where urban, semi-urban and rural peoples' livelihood have been represented.

SECTION 2: FAMILY RELATED INFORMATION OF THE RESPONDENTS

Family is the basic institutions of human civilization and this study considers it to know the psycho-social construction of the study population in order to know their behavioral pattern. Besides, it also helps to know the socialization process and links to knowledge, attitude and practices of the respondents related to COVID-19 pandemic and how they mitigate to face the disease. For understanding family nature, it captures types of family, Family head, HH sizes, children under 5 years, adult and disable members of the families.

According to Figure 3.2.1, two types of family have been identified that are nuclear and joint family by nature.

Figure 3.2.1: Types of the Family

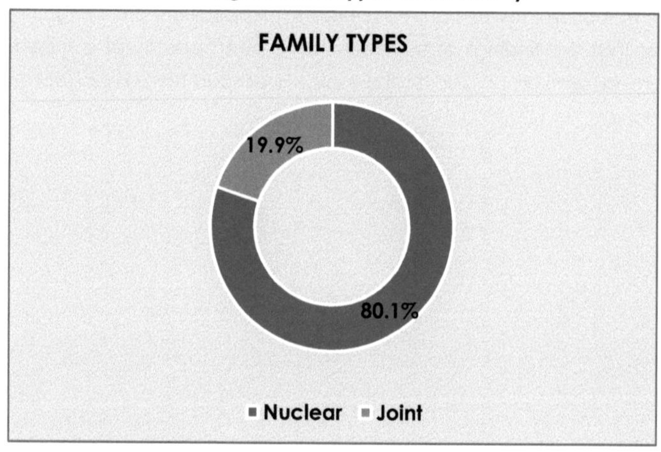

According to the information, 80.1 percent respondents have been taken from 'Nuclear family' and 19.9 percent from 'Joint family'. This information helps to understand whether any difference has been practiced between these two-family structures to mitigate the pandemic crisis and other issues. And how joint family helps each other than the nuclear family; besides, what differences are shown between urban and rural family patterns, especially for crisis mitigation during lockdown and quarantine situation, which respondents have experienced.

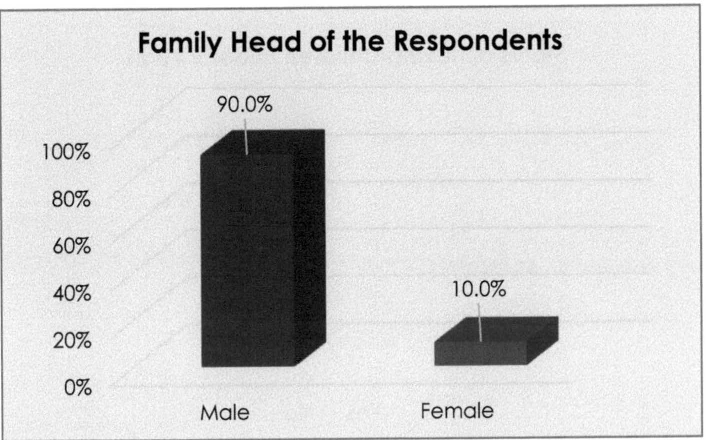

Regarding HH head, Figure 3.2.2 shows that who is HH head and it has identified, 90% are male and 10% are female who are carrying responsibilities as HH heads.

Table 3.2.1: Distribution of the household size of the participants

Family Size	n	%
Small Family (1-3 Members)	196	30.6
Medium Family (4-6 Members)	396	62.0
Large Family (>=7 Members)	47	7.4
Total	**639**	**100**

The given table 3.2.1 depicts that the size of the household of the respondents is categorized in three patterns that are `small, medium, and large family'. The family of 4-6 members called medium family which represents 62 percent, where large family is consisted 7 or more Member that represented 7.4%. But it has seen that 30.6 are small family which consisted with 1 to 3 members.

It is also considered whether the families have children who are under 5 years old for knowing whether their basic needs have been violated or not due to COVID-19. This study tries to reveal if children are faced crisis how family members cope-up with that human-crisis. And it is mandatory to protect children's right and fulfill their needs through proper taken care in proper ways. Understanding the importance, it has collected this information.

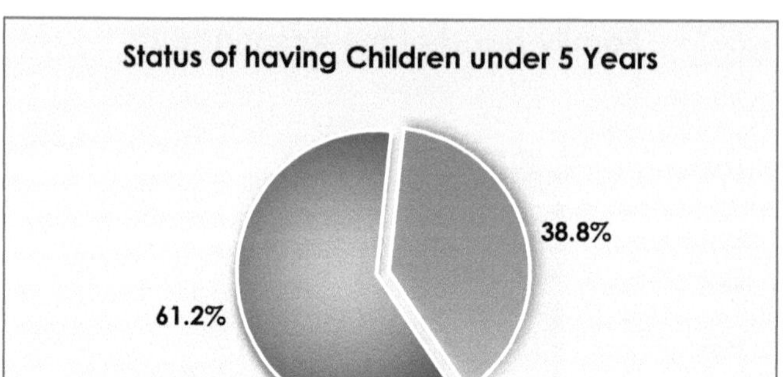

Figure 3.2.3: Status of having Children under 5 Years

And through Figure 3.2.3, it has been identified that, 61.2 percent of respondents inform they have no children whose age under 5 years old but rest of 38.8 percent informed, 'they have children whose age under 5 years'. This means majority percent of the respondents do not have children under 5 years in the study area.

Same consideration has been initiated for knowing the numbers of the families where adult members are living. Here 'adult is not considered as 'life-cycle' of respondent's physiological stage only but it inquiries how it impacts on psycho-social behavioral pattern and positively play role in public-health issues like COVID-19 prevention and mitigation.

Table 3.2.2: Status of having Adult Members in the Family

Status	n	%
Yes	134	21.0
No	505	79.0
Total	639	100

Table 3.2.2 illustrates the status of having adult members in the family, where it is seen, 79 percent respondents claim that they have no adult family members whereas 21 percent have adult family members. This information tries to make a correlation between those families who have adult members and using pandemic preventive measures, mitigation approaches and impact of livelihood and so on than the families where no adult member(s). And whether it bears any significance or not, when one family faced pandemic like COVID-19 without adult members.

Disable persons have been always taken concentration much, due to their illness or abnormal syndrome, physically and psychologically both and which differs them from the people who have normal physique. During COVID-19, what types of problems they have faced which families have disable persons and how vulnerable they are or not than the families where no disable persons.

Figure 3.2.4: Status of having any Members with Disability in the Family

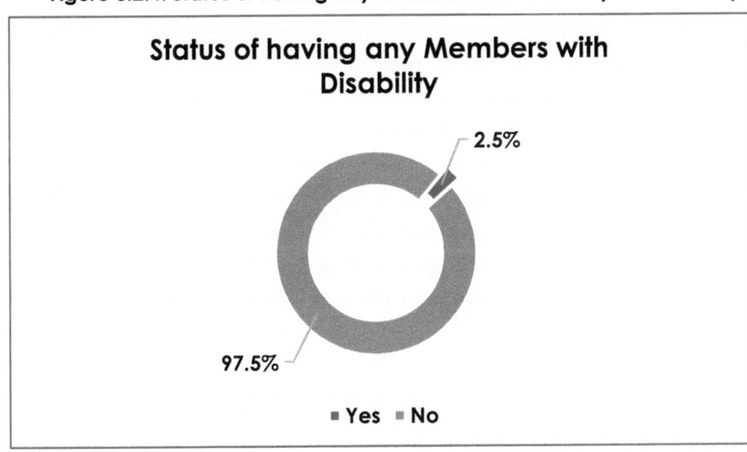

In this regard, Figure 3.2.4 contains the status of family members of disability. According to the collected data, 97.5 percent of respondents' family have no disable members but only 2.5 percent respondents' families have disable family members. Based on the information, the numbers do not have significance that influence on the whole mitigation process against COVID-19.

If it could be made a conclusion based on family related information that has importance in this rapid assessment in consideration to how family structure helps to face the challenges of COVID-19 and have any learnings from nuclear or joint family, in this regard. And which family structure and kinship pattern enable to the family-members to face any Pandemic originated problems and crisis. This rapid assessment has tried to search the answer throughout the study and if any learning been identified, that a praiseworthy innovation, undoubtedly.

SECTION 3: RESPONDENT'S KNOWLEDGE ABOUT NOVEL CORONAVIRUS

Knowledge, Attitude and Practice (KAP) is considered as basic way to explore the objectives of the assessment to understand the respondent's psychological and behavioral pattern that response towards COVID-19. One of basic thrusts to analysis, what the knowledge level of the study population has and how they practice in comparison to the knowledge. Considering it, this study has exaggerated all these issues in detail in the following sections.

Figure 3.3.1: Status of Knowing the transmission process of Novel Corona Virus of Respondents

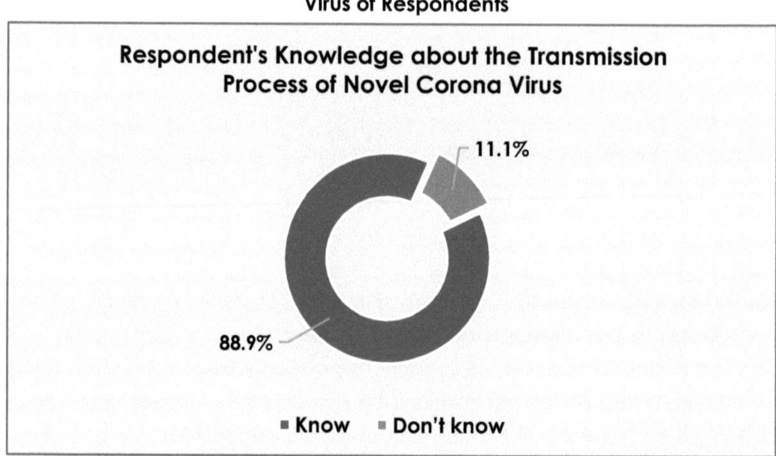

Figure 3.3.1 illustrates the status of knowing transmission process of Novel Corona Virus of the respondents. For this, 639 respondents have been interviewed for giving information about its transmission process. It has seen, 88.9 percent (n=568 out of 639 respondents) claims that they have been informed how transmission process of COVID-19 working for and another 11.1 percent of the respondents do not know about the transmission process of Novel Corona Virus.

Regarding means of Corona Virus transmission, that is very important component for this study and relevant information has been collected from the respondents. The given table 3.3.1 demonstrates that how novel corona virus has been spreading among one to other based on respondents' opinion. According to the collected information, three techniques have become indispensable for transmission.by contact with contaminated surfaces (34.3 percent), talking closely to someone infected (25.1 percent), and through the air (21.6 percent)' and these are the highest figures.

Table 3.3.1: Respondent's opinion about means of Corona Virus can transmission*
(N= 568)

Transmission Process	%
By contact with contaminated surfaces (From the sneeze / cough / phlegm / cold / spit of the infected person)	34.3
Talking closely to someone infected (respiratory droplets)	25.1
Through the Air	21.6
By providing hygiene care to infected people	13.1
By consuming contaminated food or water	1.9
By sexual contact	2.1
By insect bites	1.5
By Others way	0.4
Total	**100**

Multiple answers

On the other hand, another few means has been identified for transmitting as like 'by other way (0.4%), by insect bites (1.5%), by consuming contaminated food or water (1.9%), and by providing hygiene care to infected people (13.1%).

Figure 3.3.2: Status of having knowledge about the symptoms of COVID-19

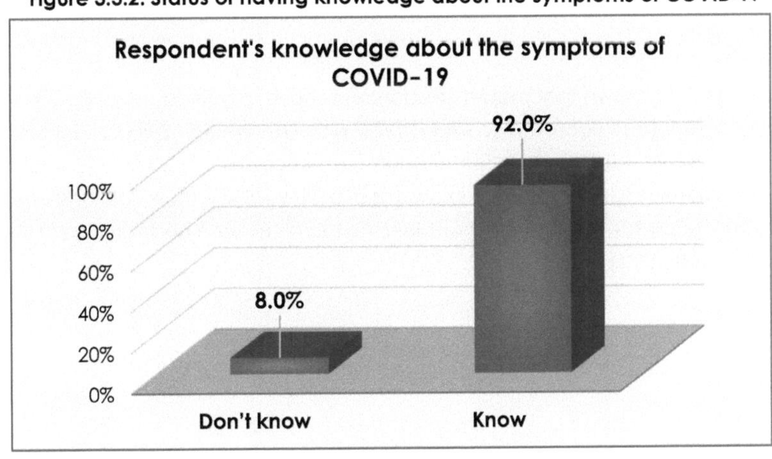

When it has been searched 'status of having knowledge about the symptom of COVID-19'; the figure 3.3.2 presents that 92 percent of them claim that they know about the symptoms whereas 8 percent do not know about the symptoms of COVID-19.

How many types of symptoms been identified, table 3.3.2 represents that there are eleven categories symptoms that they have identified namely headache, loss of smell, shortness of breath, fever, sore muscles, fatigue, bleeding, nausea and vomiting, diarrhea, cough, and sore throat. (see table 3.3.2)

Table 3.3.2: Major Symptoms of COVID-19 Considered by the Respondents*
(N=588)

Types of Symptoms	%
Headache	9.7
Loss of smell	0.6
Shortness of breath	23.7
Fever	29.7
Sore Muscles	1.5
Fatigue	1.0
Bleeding	0.1
Nausea and vomiting	0.8
Diarrhea	2.6
Cough	13.6
Sore throat	16.8
Total	**100**

Multiple answers

And it has known that majority respondents have identified 'fever (29.7 percent), and 'shortness of breath problem' (23.7 percent) where 16.8 percent identified, 'sore throat and 13.6 percent `cough' as symptoms of COVID-19. Additionally, every few respondents have knowledge on these symptoms 'loss of smell (0.6%), sore muscles (1.5%), fatigue (1%), bleeding (0.1%), nausea and vomiting (0.8%), and diarrhea (2.6%) respectively.

Another important matter is after how many days these symptoms will be appeared when someone infected with Corona.

Figure 3.3.3: Opinion of the Respondents about the symptoms appear after how many days later of infection

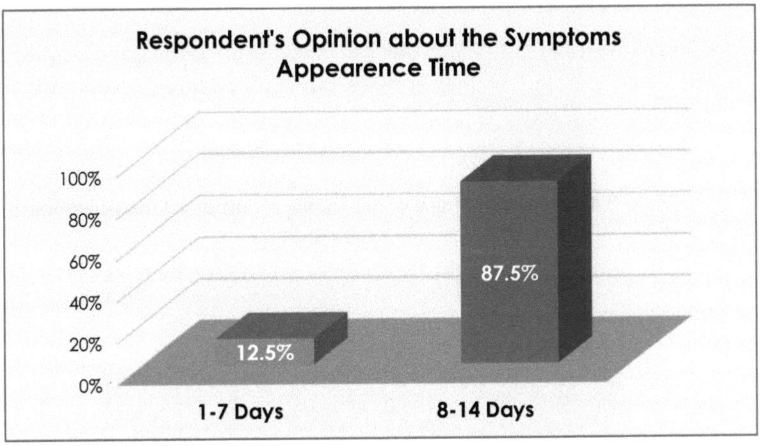

The given figure 3.3.3 depicts that 87.5% respondents have said, symptoms will appear within 8-14 days after having infection and 12.5% has mentioned, 'within 1-7 days after infection.

As the discussed information, it has seen most of the respondents have knowledge regarding Corona virus related issues as like symptoms and transmission process. This identification helps us to understand a community who have good knowledge on COVID-19 that is applicable for the study community situated at Bogura district town and adjacent areas, the Northern Region of Bangladesh.

SECTION 4: INFECTION OF CORONAVIRUS AMONG THE FAMILY MEMBERS AND NEIGHBORS

This study has collected information on Corona infected family members and neighbors. And these figures help to understand, how numbers have been infected and which role they have played to control it or not. So, it has huge importance in this study to make correlation between knowledge and practices among the numbers of infected family members.

According to the table (3.4.1), 91.5 percent of the respondents have claimed, `no' one has been infected of their families but 8.5% informed, `yes, their family members been infected'.

Table 3.4.1: Infection Status of the family members of the respondent by COVID-19

Status	n	%
Yes	54	8.5
No	585	91.5
Total	**639**	**100**
Types of Infected Person		
Respondent Himself	11	20.4
Spouse	8	14.8
Child	2	3.7
Parents	8	14.8
Brother/Sister	6	11.1
Others*	19	35.2
Total	**54**	**100**

*Others including Grand Father/Mothers, Uncle/Aunt, Cousin.

Regarding types of infected persons; according to the table 5.1, there are six categories of family members have been identified among whom 20.4 percent 'respondent himself, 14.8% 'spouse, 3.7% children, 14.8% parents and 11.1% brother and sisters have been infected. But it has mentioned 35.2% `other' that includes Grand Father/Mothers, Uncle/Aunt and Cousin.

Figure 3.4.1: Infection Status of the neighbor of the respondent by COVID-19

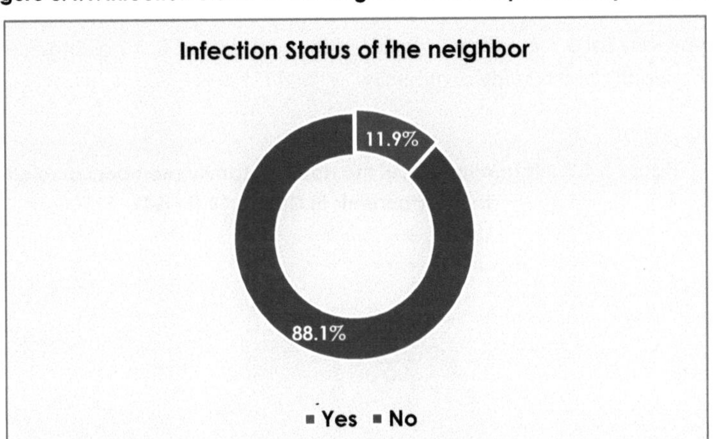

The above figure 3.4.1 represents the infection status of the neighbor of the participants regarding COVID-19 and it is seen that 88.1 percent claimed `no neighbor' of them are infected but 11.9 percent respondents claimed, their neighbor has been infected by COVID-19. This indicates, neighbors are less infected than the respondent's own family members.

Table 3.4.2: Status of having close connection of Respondent's family with COVID-19 infected neighbors

Status	n	%
Yes	7	9.2
No	69	90.8
Total	76	100

The table 3.4.2. states that the status of having close collection to the respondent's family with Novel Corona Virus infected neighbor and it is revealed that 69 participants out of total 76 participants (90.8 percent of all) have 'no' intimate connection with those neighbors who infected by COVID-19. Rest of the respondents (9.2 percent of total 76 respondents) have somehow connection with COVID-19 infected neighbors. Therefore, it has seen majority percent of the respondent's families have no connection with other infected neighbors of COVID-19.

Globally many people have been died due to COVID-19 pandemic and many are suffering till now also. And meanwhile, millions of people have been withered away irrespective of all countries since immediate spreading of this virus. And to know the morbidity ratio is important for this study, and probably it has projected the death scenario of the study community.

Figure 3.4.2: Information about the death of family members or relatives of the respondents in COVID-19 (N=54)

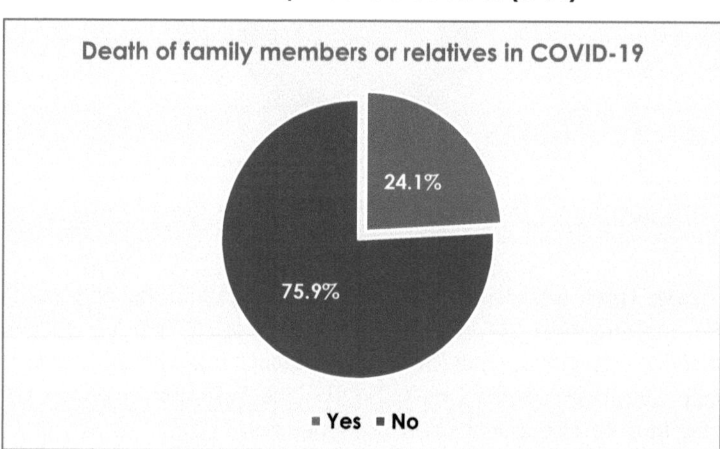

Considering this, Figure 3.4.2 shows the information about the death ratio of family members as well as relatives of the respondents in COVID-19. Among the infected family member of the respondents (54 out of 639) 75.9 percent has answered 'No' which means not a single family member or relative has been died due to COVID-19. But 24% of them says 'Yes' (13 respondents out of 54) which means respondent's family members or relatives have been died due to COVID-19.

Based on this, it is indicated, 13 persons were died among the 54 infected family members or respondents themselves. Though the figure is counted small but the rate of morbidity is 24 percent that is alarming enough.

SECTION 5: PREVENTIVE MEASURES PRACTICED BY THE RESPONDENTS

This is one of important issues that have indicated the gap between knowledge and practice that the respondents followed to mitigate the targeted disease. To understand this, present study captures various measures of World Health Organization (WHO) and National Guideline that advocated for Corona protection and control. Regarding in assessing the practices status of them, the following tables explain what frequencies of the study population have practiced the measures or not through four categories 'rarely practice, sometimes practice, often practice and Always practice'. The following tables explain these important measures that is highly helpful to understand the behavioral pattern of any community.

Table 3.5.1: Frequency of hand washing or using hand sanitizer in last three days of survey-

Hand Washing Status	Rarely (0%-25% of the time)		Sometimes (26%-50% of the time)		Often (51%-75% of the time)		Always (76%-100% of the time)		Total	
	n	%	n	%	n	%	n	%	n	%
After taking off mask	114	17.8	256	40.1	240	37.6	29	4.5	639	100
After coughing or sneezing	173	27.1	247	38.7	163	25.5	56	8.8	639	100
After returning home from outside	125	19.6	159	24.9	232	36.3	123	19.2	639	100
Average %	21.5%		34.6%		33.1%		10.8%			

Table 3.5.1 depicts the frequency of washing hand by using sanitizer since last three days period of time and for assessing this, three behavioral habits have been considered namely 'After taking off mask', 'After coughing or sneezing' and 'After returning home from outside'. When it has identified how many respondents used hand sanitizer after taking off mask, as collected information, only 4.5 percent respondents using hand sanitizer 'Always' (100% time) where all respondents have practiced it partially that considered as Rarely (0-25% of the time), Sometimes (26-50% of the time) and Often (51-75% of the time) that represents 17.8%, 40.1% and 37.6% of the using-time.

Regarding after coughing or sneezing, only 8.8 percent have practiced it 'always' but other 88.2% respondents did not use it all time that means they have used it from 0-75% time which categorized here 'as Rarely (0-25% of the time), Sometimes (26-50% of the time) and Often (51-75% of the time) (for detail, see the table 3.5.1). The picture is relatively better regarding 'after returning home from outside' that indicated 19.2% 'Always', 19.6% Rarely, 24.9% Sometimes and Often 36.3%.

That means the practice status is less than the knowledge ratio which they claimed on protective measures. Now if it is assessed average percentage that represents for three types of practices are 21.5% rarely, 34.6% sometimes, 33.1% often and 10.8% always. And it should have opportunity for THS to develop awareness program in this regard with community people.

This is another type of important measure that is 'using soap or hand wash for hand washing' in last 3 days since data collection.

Table 3.5.2: Frequency of using soap/hand wash for washing hands in last three days

Frequency	n	%
Rarely (0%-25% of the time)	80	12.5
Sometimes (26%-50% of the time)	168	26.3
Often (51%-75% of the time)	284	44.4
Always (76%-100% of the time)	107	16.7
Total	639	100

According to the Table 3.5.2, only 16.7% have practiced it 'always' but other respondents did not use it all the time that means they use it from 0-75% time which represented' 12.5% 'Rarely, 26.3% Sometimes and 44.4 % Often, (for detail, see the table 3.5.2). That indicates, a large number of respondents do not have practice soap/hand wash for washing hands 'though they have the knowledge, as claimed.

Time duration spending for washing the hands is also important for knowing the practice habit of the respondents that is highly related to protect corona virus infection. And as per WHO guideline, 20 seconds is minimum time for hand washing in order to disinfection. Understanding the importance, this study has collected the related information.

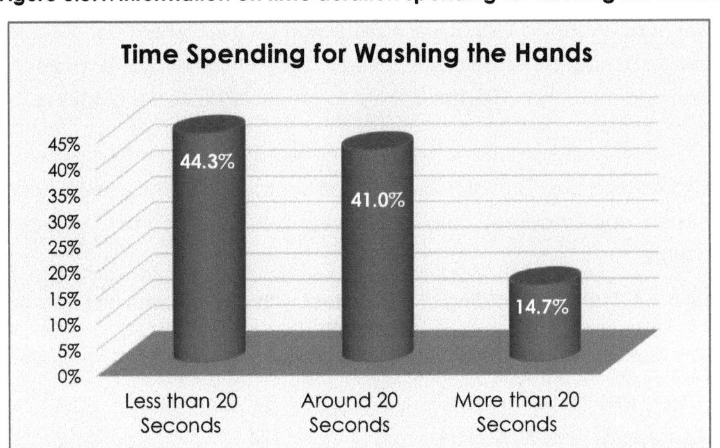

And the given figure represents the information regarding spending time of washing hands listed as 'less than 20 seconds', 'around 20 seconds', and 'more than 20 seconds'. And it is seen, 44.3 percent of the respondents spent 'less than 20 seconds' for washing hands which is highest and 41 percent respondents used 'around 20 seconds' at the moment of washing hands and 14.7 percent used 'more than 20 seconds' for washing hands. The important identification is 44% do not practice '20 second time' for hand washing as the health guideline of WHO and this is gap between knowledge and practice.

This is another type of approach that is practiced for protecting Corona infection.

Table 3.5.3: Status of Covering Mouth and Nose by hand/Elbow/Tissue paper when coughing or Sneezing

Frequency	n	%
Rarely (0%-25% of the time)	168	26.3
Sometimes (26%-50% of the time)	240	37.5
Otten (51%-75% ot the time)	173	27.1
Always (76%-100% of the time)	58	09.1
Total	639	100

The above-mentioned table (3.5.3) illustrates the status of covering mouth and nose by using hand or elbow or tissue paper at the time of coughing or sneezing where the number of total 639 participants is categorized in four patterns namely 'rarely (0 to 25 percent of the time), sometimes (26 to 50 percent of the time), often (51 to 75 percent of the time), and always (76 to 100 percent of the time)'. It has been seen only 9.1 percent have practiced it 'always' that the lowest ratio where 37.5 percent respondents practiced it 'sometimes'. In this regard, another 27.1

percent have claimed they practiced it 'often (51% to 75% of the time) and 26.3 percent as rarely (0% to 25% of the time). Based on this figure, it has revealed that very few respondents (9.1 percent) have practiced this 'always' for protecting the infection and more than 90% have failed to practice this as per guideline.

Table 3.5.4 shows the status of avoiding close contact with anyone who has a fever and cough, and it has seen, only 16.3% have avoid close contact who has fever and cough'.

Table 3.5.4: Status of avoiding close contact with anyone who has a fever and cough

Frequency	n	%
Rarely (0%-25% of the time)	88	13.8
Sometimes (26%-50% of the time)	174	27.2
Often (51%-75% of the time)	273	42.7
Always (76%-100% of the time)	104	16.3
Total	**639**	**100**

Here it is seen that 42.7 percent respondents are the highest who practiced it 'often' and 27.2 percent 'sometimes'. But 13.8 percent respondents practiced it 'rarely (0 to 25 percent of the time)'. Now if it is calculated that total numbers who do not practice 'always' that is more than 80% who do not avoid close contact with anyone who has a fever and cough.

The following figure 3.5.2 represents the status of wearing face mask at the time of outdoor activities like attending office, doing market and other activities.

Figure 3.5.2: Status of wearing face mask when stay in outside of home

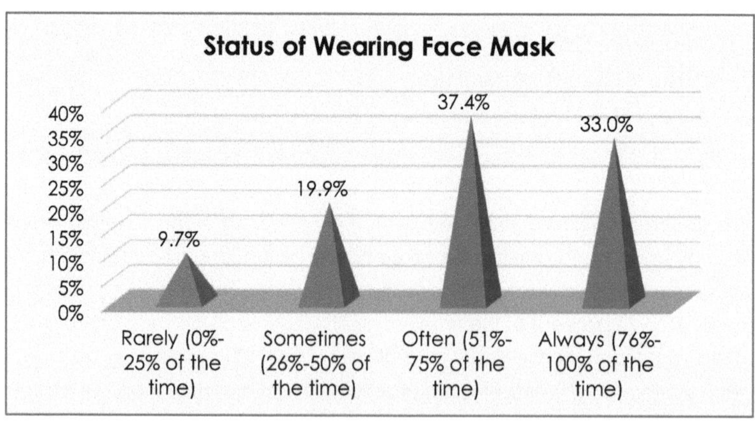

It is observed that 33 percent of total respondents have worn face mask 'always' (76% to 100% of the time) when they stay in outside of home but rest of them that means 77% respondents do not use or regularly use the mask when they outside of home. Through this, though it is found maximum percent of total respondents is aware in terms of wearing face mask at outdoor activities but not 'always' that will be advised to wear face mask at outdoor activities by the medical guideline.

Regarding status of maintaining social distance is very important for protecting COVID-19 and it is mostly advised by the concerned authority to the mass people to follow. So, it is considered as important issue and this study has collected information on how the respondents practice it or not in their daily lives.

Table 3.5.5: Status of maintaining social distance when stay in outside of home

Frequency	n	%
Rarely (0%-25% of the time)	200	31.3
Sometimes (26%-50% of the time)	234	36.6
Often (51%-75% of the time)	151	23.6
Always (76%-100% of the time)	54	8.5
Total	639	100

According to the table 3.5.5, only 8.5% respondents have maintained social distance 'always' but rest of the respondents 91.5% have failed to follow it all time. As table, it has known, 36.6 percent respondents practice it 'sometimes' (26 percent to 50 percent of the time) and 31.3% percent practiced it 'rarely' and 23.3 percent 'often'. In overall, it may be said most of the respondents' maintained social distance 'partially' and only 8.5% 'always'.

Regarding the status of taking a body shower soon after returning home from outside and it is seen 11.7% have it 'always' properly whereas 29.6% took shower 'rarely' after back home from outside.

Table 3.5.6: Status of taking a body Shower soon after returning home from outside

Frequency	n	%
Rarely (0%-25% of the time)	189	29.6
Sometimes (26%-50% of the time)	210	32.9
Often (51%-75% of the time)	165	25.8
Always (76%-100% of the time)	75	11.7
Total	639	100

But 29.6 percent practiced it 'rarely' and 32.9 percent and 32.9 percent informed that they practiced it 'sometimes'.

According to the related information, the status of taking shower after returning home from outdoor activities is not practiced all time though they have the knowledge.

Regarding preventive measure practice, 'staying at home without any emergency' is another behavior that need to be followed by the people.

Figure 3.5.3: Status of staying at home without any emergency

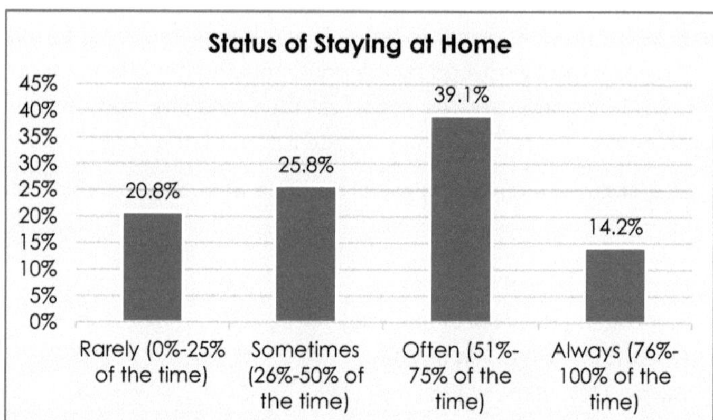

The figure 5.3.3 has illustrated that only 14% respondents have followed 'always' 'staying at home without emergency' but rest of the respondents have informed 'rarely' (21%), 'sometimes' (26%) and 'often' (39%). That means 86% respondents do not staying at home all time though general norms that need to be followed.

Based on above discussion, it has informed that no measure has been followed always (100%) by all the respondents. Though when they have asked about knowledge of the preventive measures, they informed they have the knowledge. Regarding gap identification between knowledge and practice, huge gap has been found in practice.

SECTION 6: INFORMATION SOURCES OF COVID-19

In knowing the sources and accessibility to the sources of information both are important in relation to Individual and social aspects where respondents have been living. Because, if people have no easy access to sources where the relevant COVID-information are available, how possible for community to response towards COVID-19 appropriately. This section tries to explain this critical issue that directly enhance people's knowledge and idea for health-related issues and identify how many have no access to information though both are living in same community.

In this regard, three sources are taken under consideration these are 'Accessibility to awareness on prevention and other crucial information about Covid-19, Key Sources of Information for Respondents on COVID-19, Opinion of the Respondents about having the knowledge for preventing COVID-19 and Opinion of the Respondents about having the knowledge for preventing COVID-19.

Table 3.6.1: Accessibility to sources of awareness on prevention and other crucial information about Covid-19

Accessibility	n	%
Can fully access to information	345	54.0
Can partially access to information	272	42.6
Cannot access to information	22	03.4
Total	639	100

Regarding accessibility to sources of awareness on prevention and other crucial information about COVID-19; it has seen that 54 percent respondents have informed 'can fully access to information' and 42.6% have 'partial access to information' in knowing COVID and its prevention. However, 3.4 percent respondents informed, they have 'no access to information' that helps them to raising awareness regarding these issues. Data has been shown that though the figure of 'fully and partially' accessibility are good but few have fully out of circle in in this regard (03.4%).

Regarding sources of information, table 3.6.2. represents seven types of sources have been identified includes electronic and print media like TV, Radio, Newspaper, Non-Government workers, Neighbors, Relatives and Friends, Health workers, Leaflet or Miking, Social media and Religious leaders.

Table 3.6.2: Key Sources of Information for Respondents on COVID-19

Key Sources	Yes		No	
	n	%	n	%
Electronics and Print Media (TV, Radio, News Paper)	504	78.9	135	21.1
NGO Workers	387	60.6	252	39.4
Neighbors, Relatives & Friends	281	44.0	358	56.0
Health Workers	255	39.9	384	60.1
Leaflet/Miking	158	24.7	481	75.3
Social Media	144	22.5	495	77.5
Religious Leaders	68	10.6	571	89.4

*Multiple answer

And most the effective sources that have been used are 'Electronics and Print Media (TV, Radio, News Paper) (78.9%), NGO Workers (60.6%), Neighbors, Relatives & Friends (44%) and Health workers (39.9%)'. In addition, as sources of information, 24.7% respondents used 'Leaflet/Miking, 22.5% used 'social media' and 10.6% 'religious leaders'. Regarding the sources of information, it is made conclusion, electronic, print media and social medias have been used mostly by the respondents as sources in getting information on COVID-19.

Figure 3.6.1 depicts that the opinion of the respondents about having the knowledge for preventing COVID-19. It is observed that 63.1 percent respondents give the statement 'Yes' which means majority number (63.1 percent) of the respondents has sufficient knowledge for preventing this COVID-19 pandemic.

Figure 3.6.1: Opinion of the Respondents about having the knowledge for preventing COVID-19

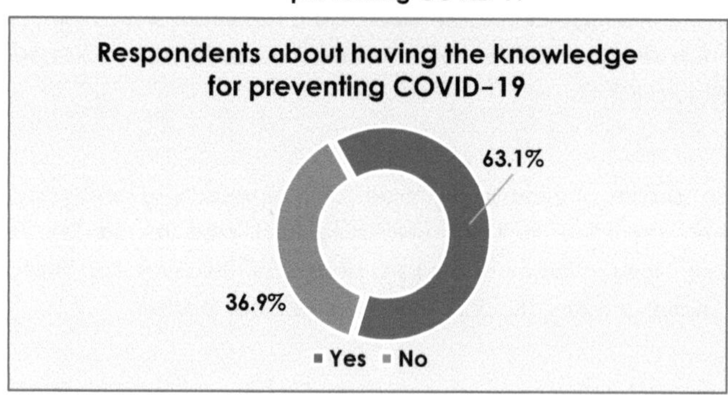

Whereas 36.9 percent respondents said 'No' which means that those respondents have 'partial knowledge' for preventing COVID-19.

46

This is very important that which measures need to be taken for enhancing the respondents' knowledge in order to protecting COVID-19. As collected suggestions given by the respondents (n=236) (Table 3.6.3) namely 'special awareness campaign (19.9%), courtyard meeting (44.5%), Miking (28.8%), and poster/leaflet and flyer (6.8%)'. In this regard, 236 people have been taken as study respondent for conducting survey.

Table 3.6.3: Measure need to be taken for enhancing the knowledge of Respondents about COVID-19

Measures	n	%
Special awareness campaign can be organized	47	19.9
Courtyard Meeting can be organized	105	44.5
Miking can be increased	68	28.8
Poster/leaflet/flyer distribution can be increased	16	6.8
Total	236	100

Based on collected suggestion, all the measures need to be taken for enhancing peoples' knowledge for preventing COVID-19 pandemic. And for taking new awareness program, TMSS Health Section (THS)Authority should have consider this among their beneficiaries and community people.

SECTION 7: IMPACT OF COVID-19 ON LIVELIHOOD, INCOME AND FOOD IN-TAKE

Whatever the status of knowledge and practice of the community people, another important objective of this study that needs to be analyzed how impact COVID-19 on the people's livelihood in respect to various considerations including income, food-taking, treatment, transportation and so on. Information has been available locally, regionally and globally on these issues that indicated COVID-19 impacts badly on people's livelihood irrespective of countries and continents. This study has made good effort to know how COVID-19 impacts in a specific community in northern Bangladesh and in which extent. Another important matter has been untapped, how local people have cope-up with the situation and through which means. Explanation have been made in the succeeding sections that helps to understand the whole situation which clarifies livelihood crisis and mitigation approaches that people have practiced and how community played role in this regard or not.

Figure 3.7.1: Status of affecting households' livelihoods due to the COVID-19 Pandemic

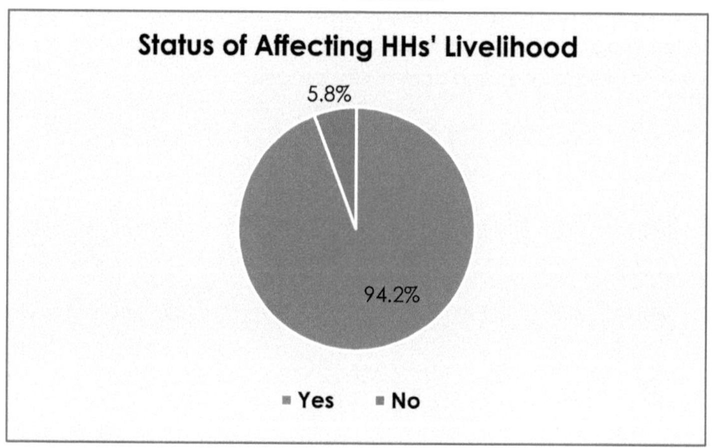

Figure 3.7.1 represents the status of affecting households' (HH) livelihood due to COVID-19 pandemic. According to the information, 94.20 percent respondents informed, their HH livelihood have been affected due to COVID-19 pandemic and out of 5.80 percent claimed 'did not affected'.

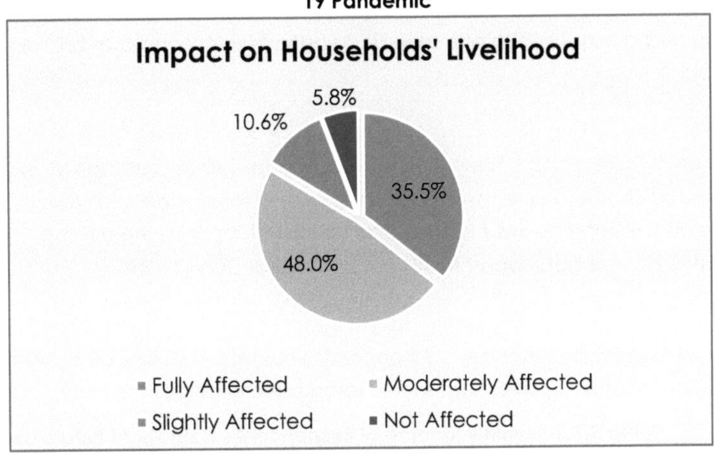

And those have been affected (As Figure 3.7.2) in what extent, 48% is the highest ratio that have been affected in 'moderately' whereas 35.5% 'fully affected'. In this regard, 10.60% have been affected 'slightly'; on the contrary 5.80%. are identified as 'not affected'. In short, it is commented about 94% respondents' HHs have been affected more or less during COVID-19 which shrinks their basic facilities during the study period.

Question is what types of change have been seen pre and during COVID-19; according to the table, 3.7.1. it has known that most of the respondents' occupation have been change during COVID-19.

Table 3.7. 1: Major Source of Income of Respondent's household Pre and during onset of COVID-19

Income (BDT)	Pre-COVID-		During COVID	
	n	%	n	%
Salary	140	21.9	95	14.9
Daily/Casual Laborer	122	19.1	101	15.8
Agriculture/Livestock	214	33.5	203	31.8
Own Business	112	17.5	99	15.5
Others Profession	44	6.9	43	6.7
Support from Family/Relative/Friends	5	0.8	26	4.1
Social Safety-net	0	0.0	47	7.4
No Income	2	0.3	25	3.9
Total	639	100	639	100

It affects mostly on agriculture and livestock that is pre-33.5 and during 31.8 (see the table 3.7.2) percent and next is daily and casual labor which reflects pre-19.1 and during post 15.8%. It also seen decreasing of salary and own business (see the table.

When it is searched how they have mitigated their decreased income; as information, they have taken support from their family and relatives which is pre-COVID 0.8% and during 4.1% however safety net supports them mostly that is pre-COVID no one get support (0.0%) but and during COVID 7.4%.

Regarding monthly income of respondent's household before and during COVID-19 (See table-3.7.2) and it has seen average decreasing of the income ceiling.

Table 3.7.2: Monthly income of Respondent's Household Before and During onset of COVID-19

Income (BDT)	Before COVID-19		During COVID-19		Changes	
	n	%	n	%	n	%
≤10000	184	28.8	428	67.0	+244	+38.2
10001-20000	266	41.6	166	26.0	-100	-15.6
20001-30000	113	17.7	32	5.0	-81	-12.7
30001-40000	40	6.3	06	0.9	-34	-5.4
40001-50000	26	4.1	05	0.8	-21	-3.3
>50000	10	1.6	02	0.3	-06	-1.3
Total	639	100.0	639	100.0		
Average Income	19536.00 BDT		10638.00 BDT		-8898.00 BDT	

And respondents' HH income ceiling been decreased '-15.6% whose income 10001-20000 and another category is 20001-30000 -12.7%'. Another concern issue is that 38.2 percent respondents' income have been reduced during COVID-19 and now they belong in income group ≤10,000 BDT.

Regarding experiencing the problems due to faced COVID-19; Figure 3.7.3 represents that 88.7 percent respondents who have experienced income drop due to this pandemic which is the highest, and 7% respondents who have lost their jobs during COVID-19 the lowest figure.

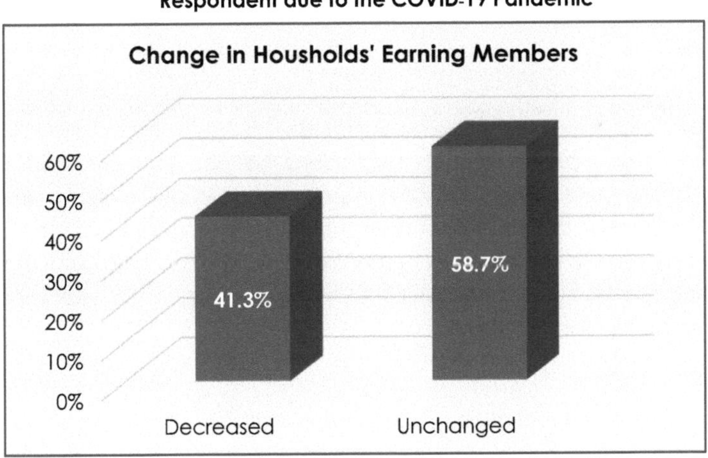

But those who have lost access to markets to sell production, those who have closed shop or market, and who have lost their livelihood money are 34.7 percent, 29.1 percent and 22.7 percent respectively. That means all types of earning source have been decreased due to COVID lockdown and people have suffered a lot for that.

Figure 3.7.4: Status of Changing in Household's Earning Members of the Respondent due to the COVID-19 Pandemic

Beyond this, the given figure 3.7.4 shows 'the status of changing-household's earning members of the respondents due to COVID-19 pandemic; according to the figure, it is seen, majority number (41.3 percent) of the earning members have been faced income decreasing whereas 58.7 percent claims that their number of households-earning members have been unchanged. The scenario is relatively good though families income have been decreased in total.

Expenditure depends on income and table 3.7.3 represents monthly expenditure of respondent's household before and during of COVID-19 and it has identified all types of income group have experienced decreased their income during COVID-19. And as information, whose monthly expenditure are 10001 to 15000 BDT that decreased for 7.5% respondents and it has known most of the highest income groups have faced expenditure decreasing from 15001-more than 30000 BDT (see the table 3.7.3 for detail).

Table 3.7.3: Monthly Expenditure of Respondent's Household before and after onset of COVID-19

Expenditure (BDT)	Before COVID		During COVID		Changes	
	n	%	n	%	n	%
≤5000	66	10.3	114	17.8	+45	+7.5
5001-10000	219	34.3	277	43.3	+58	+9.0
10001-15000	156	24.4	108	16.9	-48	-7.5
15001-20000	85	13.3	88	13.8	+03	+0.5
20001-25000	53	8.3	28	4.4	-25	-3.9
25001-30000	36	5.6	13	2.0	-23	-3.6
>30000	24	3.8	11	1.7	-13	-2.1
Total	639	100	639	100.0		
Average Expenditure	15598.00 BDT		11458.00 BDT		-4140 BDT	

The average expenditure of the respondents has also decreased from 15598 to 11458 before and during of COVID19 respectively and the difference is almost 4140 BDT on average for every respondent. The study also revealed that the number of respondents with comparatively higher expenditure capacity (10001 to more) has been decreased during the COVID-19 and they belong into the lower expenditure group (10 thousand or below).

Table 3.7.4 illustrates that how households are coping with the income disruption due to COVID-19 pandemic. Here, it is seen that major adaptation with income disruption as being mitigating 'quantity and quality meals' is 65.1 percent (n=392) out of 602, while 11.6 percent informed, they sold their jewelry and valuable assets. A good number of respondent (59.8%) have 'borrowed from relatives, neighbors and friends' whereas 48.8% informed they have 'mitigated by their previous savings' (see table-3.7.4).

Table 3.7.4: How households are coping with the income dropped due to COVID-19 Pandemic*

Coping Strategies	Yes		No	
	n	%	n	%
Borrowing from relatives/neighbors/friends	360	59.8	242	40.2
Loan from Informal Institutions/local CBO	90	15.0	512	85.0
Sold Jewelry or Valuable Assets	70	11.6	532	88.4
Used Savings	294	48.8	308	51.2
Reducing quantity and quality of meals	392	65.1	210	34.9

*Multiple answers

Table 3.7.5 represents the status of having three meals per day of respondents' family members during COVID-19 pandemic, and it has known 84.5 percent 'have the child members who under 5 years get at least 3 meals in a day' and the scenario is good for the adult members also that is 74.8%. Out of them, 69.6 percent respondents informed, 'all the family members get at least 3 meals in a day'.

Table 3.7.5: Status of having 3 meals in a day during the COVID-19 Pandemic

	Yes		No		Total	
	n	%	n	%	n	%
Have all the family members get at least 3 meals in a day	445	69.6	194	30.4	639	100
Have the adult members of your family get at least 3 meals in a day	478	74.8	161	25.2	639	100
Have the child members ot under 5 years get at least 3 meals in a day	540	84.5	99	15.5	639	100

According to the data of this table, many of the respondents' family do struggling to manage at least three-square meals in a day during COVID-19 pandemic and the figure is 15 to 30 percent more or less (see the table 3.7.5).

Regarding knowing the food availability is one of the important components that helps us to know the status of this. Figure 3.7.5 states 'food stock of the respondent's household during COVID-19 pandemic'; it has classified into four major types namely '1 to 3 days only, 1 week only, 1 month at least, and no food stock'.

Figure 3.7.5: Food Availability of Respondent's Household during the COVID-19 Pandemic

Range of Food Stock

According to the Figure 3.7.5, it is seen that 38 percent respondents have claimed, they have `food stock for 1-3 days only which is the highest, and 11.9 percent informed `one-month food stock which is the lowest'. In addition, other 27.7 percent and 22.4 percent respondents have informed they have food stock for one week only however, 22.40% informed, they have `no food stock' during the time of COVID-19 pandemic.

This study has also tried to discover 'nature of food availability during COVID-19 pandemic'.

Table 3.7.6: Nature of Food Availability in the Household during the COVID-19 Pandemic

Status	Yes (%)	No (%)
Starch	63.26%	36.74%
Protein Rich	22.60%	77.40%
Pulse	44.75%	55.25%
Green leafy vegetables	83.10%	16.90%
Energy dense food	36.80%	63.20%
Milk products	12.90%	87.10%

According to the collected information, table 3.7.6 illustrates 83.1 percent of the respondents claim that they have taken 'green leafy vegetables which is the highest and 12.9 percent have informed 'milk products availability' which is the lowest. Another 63.26 percent of total 639 participants have enjoyed 'starch food' but 22.60 percent respondents claimed for protein food. As concluding remark, it may be said that nature of food availability that has been contained mixed scenario where major portion of respondents failed to enjoy protein (77.40%), milk product (87.10%) and pulses (55.25%) that is important for daily calorie intake.

The table 3.7.7 depicts the household 'coping strategies for food-intake during the COVID-19 pandemic and it has seen 28.3 percent of households has 'switched to less preferred but with low-cost food', while 26.5 percent of households have reduced 'the portion size of the meals' unfortunately. Another 20.6 percent of HHs has reduced the number of meals eaten in a day.

Table 3.7.7: Households Coping strategies for food intake during the COVID-19 Pandemic (N=639)*

Coping Strategies	n	%
HHs have switched to less preferred, but low-cost food	414	28.3%
HHs have reduced the portion size of the meals	388	26.5%
HHs have reduced the Number of meals eaten per day	302	20.6%
HHs have borrowed food or rely on the help from friends or relatives	119	8.1%
Adults specially Mothers have reduced the quantity of their food intake to provide for the children	78	5.3%
Families have gone through an entire day without eating	62	4.2%
Families have sent their family members to find a meal elsewhere	101	6.9%

Multiple answers

But very limited families (6.9 percent) have sent their 'family members to find a meal elsewhere', and 8.1 percent of the households whom have borrowed 'food from friends or relativos' also. In case of adapting strategies during COVID-19 pandemic, 5.3 percent of adults particularly mothers have reduced 'quantity of their food intake to provide for ensuring their children's food'. But according to the information, unfortunately, 4.2 percent of families has gone through an entire day without having any eating'.

SECTION 8: IMPACT ON ACCESSIBILITY OF ESSENTIAL HEALTH CARE SERVICES

Globally and Nationally, COVID-19 have succeeded to spread stigma and phobia that hampers people's normal lives even taking health care also. During COVID-19 situation, all over the world, health-system has been faced challenges in all aspects to provide respective health services to the people since World War-II. Questions have been raised how community people (urban, semi-urban and rural) in Bangladesh faced problem in taking any health facilities during COVID-19. In Bogura, though many health-institutes are situated both public and private in nature, but people faced challenges in getting health services both COVID-19 and other diseases. Efforts have been given to collect the information on the respondent's health services and it portraits in this section. It also helps to understand both the policy and action level strategies and it's loopholes that impact badly on the people's livelihood.

Figure 3.8.1: Status of Facing Health problems of Respondent's HHs during COVID-19

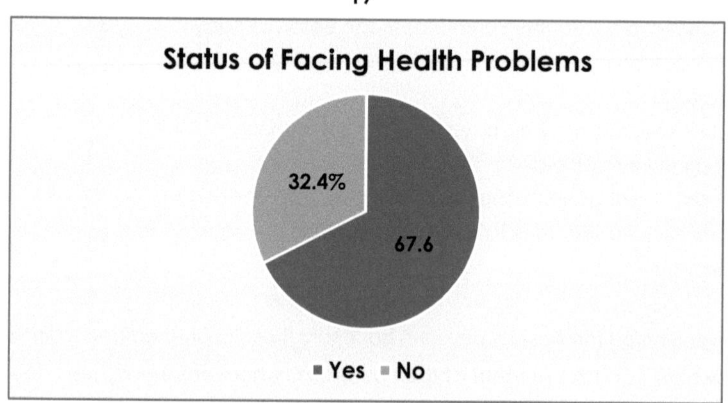

The Figure 3.8.1 shows how numbers respondents have experienced with health problems during corona virus pandemic. According to the table, where 432 respondents have claimed that their households have faced health problems during COVID-19 which is about 67.6 percent. On the other hand, only 32.4 percent respondents said 'No' they did not have faced any health problems during the pandemic.

The given figure 3.8.2 states the classifications of health problems experienced by the respondents and it has identified five categories health problems that have faced 'physical illness (24.40%), 'severe stress problems(33.10%), 'either injuries or urgent health problems (3.80), mental illness (6.30%) and respondents who faced 'no health-related problems (32.40) respectively.

Figure 3.8.2: Types of Health Problems experienced by Respondent's HHs during COVID-19

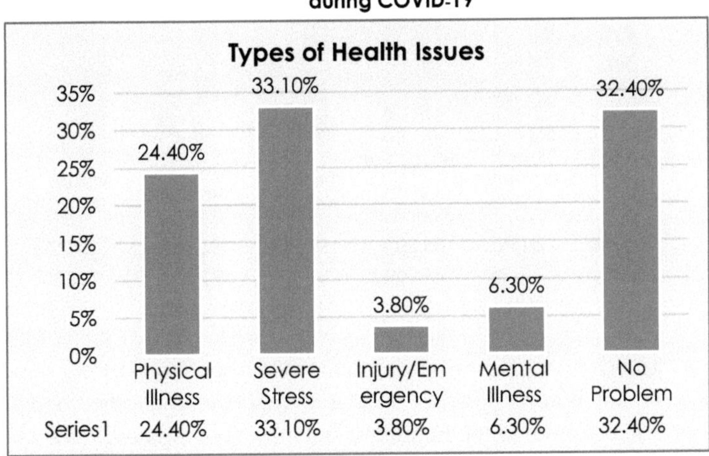

From this, it has indicated that mostly faced 'severe stress' that are 33.10% and 24.40 Percent faced 'physical illness though good information is 32.40% respondents are out of any physical illness.

The mentioned figure 3.8.3 represents the accessibility of the health institutions before and during onset of COVID-19. And it has seen that respondents have taken health services from the health institutes during COVID-19 that includes community clinic (36.84%), government hospitals (46.90%), private hospital (16.35%), traditional medicine center (52.85%), and mobile clinics (5.28). 'Regarding before taking treatment' it has seen where the highest percentage of the respondents (85.30 percent) have relied on government hospital and the lowest percentage of the respondents (33.7 percent) have taken services from Community Clinics.

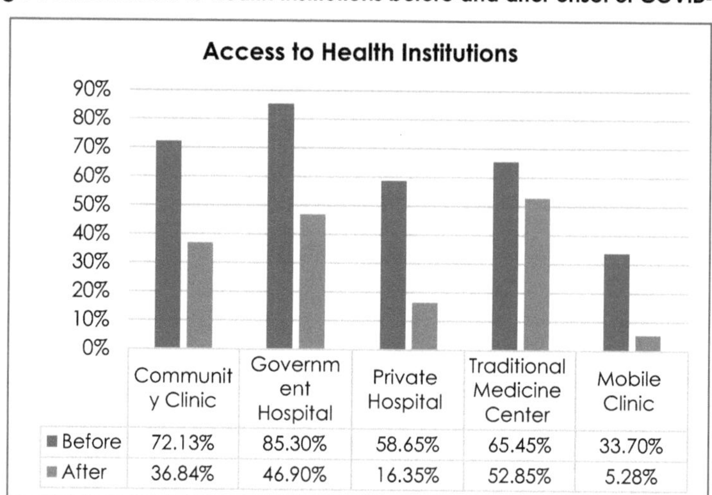

	Communit y Clinic	Governm ent Hospital	Private Hospital	Traditional Medicine Center	Mobile Clinic
■ Before	72.13%	85.30%	58.65%	65.45%	33.70%
■ After	36.84%	46.90%	16.35%	52.85%	5.28%

In a concluding remark, it may be said though the respondents mostly depended on government hospital instead of private hospitals and other health care institutions before onset of this pandemic but they have received health facilities from traditional medical centers mostly after onset of COVID-19.

Table 3.8.1: Reason behind the Low Access to Health Institutions during the COVID-19

Reasons	n	%
Due to unavailability of transport to reach at Health Institutions	180	41.7
Health Institutions was not open	32	07.4
No Doctor has presented at Health Institutions	48	11.1
Health Institutions was open but disagree to provide the service	41	09.5
Didn't go Health Institutions because of fear of getting infected by COVID-19	131	30.3
Total	432	100

Table 3.8.1 illustrates the reasons behind the low access to health institutions during novel corona virus where total 432 participants have been interviewed for this study. According to the table, 41.7 percent of the total 432 participants never took health facilities due to unavailability of transportation towards health institutions which is mark as highest, and only 7.4 percent respondents have low access to

health services due to unavailability of health institutions as lowest. But it has known that another 30.3 percent (432 respondents) did not go to health institutions due to the fear of getting infection of COVID-19. In the end it has found, respondents always do struggle to get access to health institutions during COVID-19 for taking treatment.

Figure 3.8.4 shows the status of faced problems in getting maternal and child health services of respondents' households during COVID-19.

Figure 3.8.4: Status of Facing Problems for getting Maternal and Child related Health Services of Respondent's HHs during COVID-19

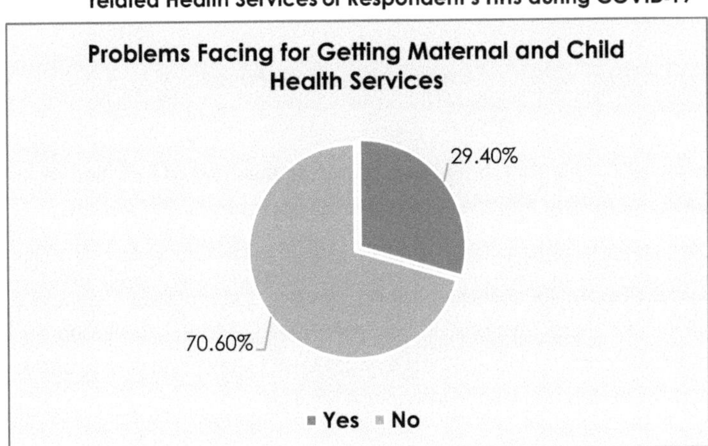

According to the information, it has been seen that 70.60 percent faced problems in getting health services for their children whereas 29.40% claimed, `no', they did not face any problem during present pandemic.

When it has searched access to health institutes for maternal and child health care, according to the figure 3.8.5, 32.9 percent respondents have said they have to accessibility to maternal and child health institutions for receiving desired services.

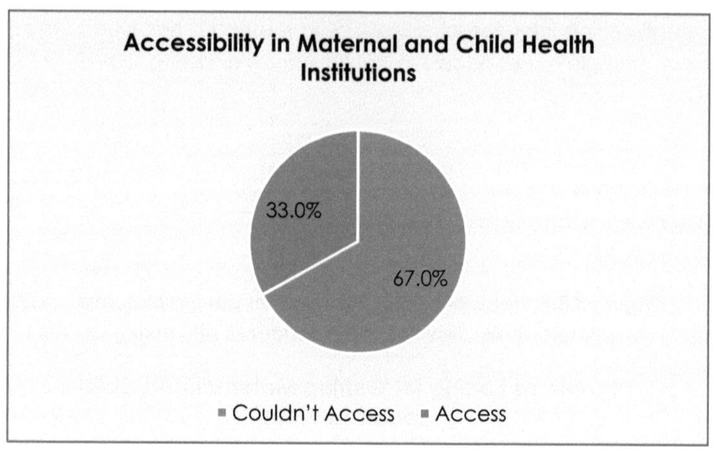

Whereas, 67.03 percent have claimed that they could not find any health institutions for getting treatment for maternal and child health services.

What the reasons for failed to taking services for maternal and children; as identified the major reasons, it has mentioned 'didn't go Health Institutions because of fear of getting infected by COVID-19 (37.4%) and Due to unavailability of transport to reach at Health Institutions (30.8%).

Table 3.8.2: Reasons of no Access to Maternal and Child Health Institutions during the COVID-19

Reasons	n	%
Due to unavailability of transport to reach at Health Institutions	39	30.8
Health Institutions was not open	07	05.6
No Doctor has presented at Health Institutions	17	13.5
Health Institutions was open but refrained from providing the service	16	12.7
Didn't go Health Institutions because of fear of getting infected by COVID-19	47	37.4
Total	126	100

But a very unconventional identification has been revealed that are 'No Doctor has presented at Health Institutions (13.5%) and Health Institutions were not open

(05.6%)'. It impacts badly in getting treatment for pregnant mother and child care also when doctors were not available in hospital or other institutes during COVID-19.

Due to COVID-19, during June-August, 2020 when this study has been conducted, lockdown was declared by the government and many types of transportation did not available on roads, even health professionals did not visit their health institutes on regular basis. The whole fact (lockdown, lack of transportation, isolation, no Doctors, policing) hampered normal health services and sometimes mothers and children have the victim of such unpredictable services.

SECTION 9: ACCESS TO HUMANITARIAN ASSISTANCE

This section of the report represents the data about the accessibility of the respondents to humanitarian assistance provided by the different types of bodies that includes Government, Non-government and other organizations during the COVID-19 period. Percentage of Accessibility, types of assistance, sources of received assistance etcetera have been discussed in this section. Which provides a clear scenario to the policy makers and government about the issue of assistance that need to be taken into account.

Figure 3.9.1: Status of receiving any types of Humanitarian assistance in COVID-19

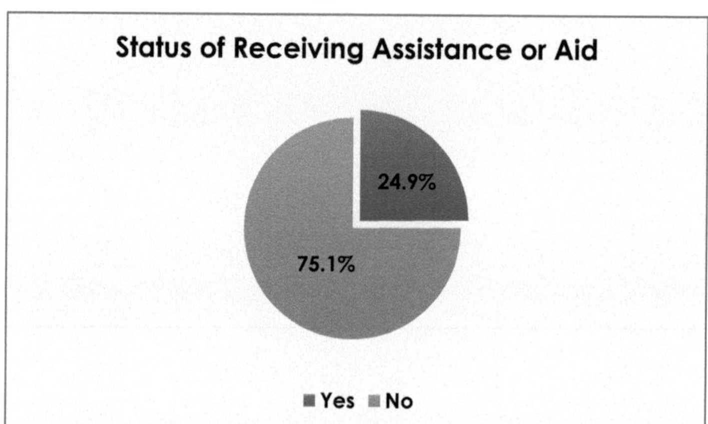

The given figure 3.9.1 depicts the status of receiving any types of assistance during COVID-19 situation especially under lockdown and quarantines, according to the information, 67.4% respondents have claimed that they have taken 'Dry Rations like Rice, Potato, Oil. etc.' and 7.8% 'different types of fruits like Apple, Orange, etc. (Fresh Food Packs),'

Table 3.9.1: Types of Assistance Received by the Respondents during COVID-19 (N=159)*

Types of Assistance	n	%
Dry Rations like Rice, Potato, Oil, etc.	147	67.4
Different types of Fruits like Apple, Orange etc. (Fresh Food Packs)	17	7.8
Money (Hand Cash, Cheque, Balance in Mobile Banking etc.)	25	11.5
Hygiene Packs like Sanitizer, Savlon, Mask etc.	21	9.6
Medicine	8	3.7
Total	**218**	**100**

Multiple Response

Whereas 11.5% have claimed that they got 'Money (Hand Cash, Cheque, Balance in Mobile Banking etc.)' as assistance. Additionally, regarding medicine (3.7%) and sanitizer (9.6%) they have got these when they are during lockdown.

Figure 3.9.2: Distribution of the Respondents by how many types of Assistance have been received by Respondents

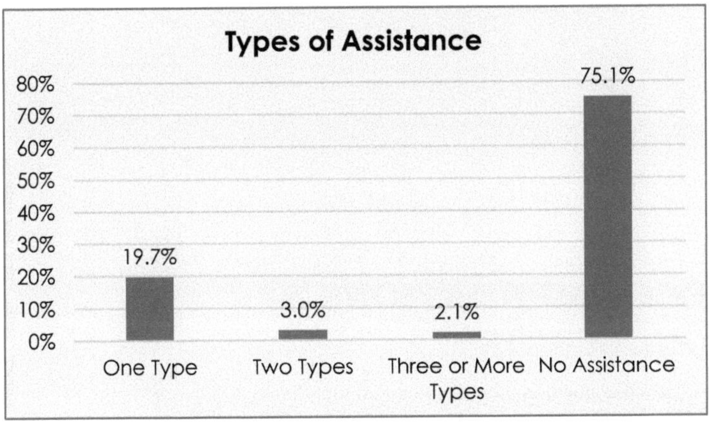

From where they have received the assistance, table 3.9.2 shows the sources of received assistance by the respondents, it has observed, respondents have taken the assistance from 'government organizations such as Union Parishad, Upazila Parishad etcetera (41.2%), NGO (39.2%), local club/institutions/societies (16.7%) and from individual people (02.9%).

Table 3.9.2: Sources of Received Assistance by the Respondents (N=159)*

Types of Assistance	n	%
Government Organizations (Union Parishad, Upazila Parishad etc.)	84	41.2
NGO	80	39.2
Local Club/Institutions/Societies	34	16.7
From Individual People	06	02.9
Total	204	100

Multiple Response

In conclusion, it may be said, through this it has been identified that more than 75% respondents taken any types of assistance including dry-food, money and sanitizers; but when it has wanted to know how many persons got more than one type assistance that is 19.70%. Besides, as agencies of distributing assistance, government and NGOs have been playing role mostly that is 41.2% and 39.2% respectively. But community engagement as like CBOs, LGIs, Clubs, Political Parties, etc. did not identified higher as like those agencies.

RECOMMENDATIONS & CONCLUSION

Conclusions

CHAPTER FOUR

CHAPTER FOUR

RECOMMENDATIONS & CONCLUSION

Screening the whole issues; many gaps and shortfalls have been identified during among the respondents, service providers and community engagements in terms of various issues. But the credibility is, many suggestions have been forwarded from the various stakeholders that helps to make recommendation for both policy and action level & these presented here as follows:

- Awareness programs should be introduced among the people on COVID-19 and its impact.
- COVID-19 test opportunities should be practiced in rural areas especially for poor people.
- Assistance and the safety-net program should be expanded during any pandemic.
- Treatment costs should be lessened or freed for corona-infected poor people.
- Alternative livelihood approach should be introduced early when lockdown be imposed.
- Health Care Institutes could be opened all time during any pandemic.
- Health Card may be introduced for the marginal people as like the safety net program.
- People should be involved personally and the community as a whole to take further steps to remove the stigma and do practices health safety rules in the COVID perspective.

CONCLUSION

During the COVID-19 pandemic situation, THS has completed a milestone Rapid Assessment to know the peoples' knowledge, prevention measures, mitigation strategy and so on of Bogura district and adjacent areas in order to identify prevention measures and mitigation strategies and so on. Through this study, several types of results have been revealed where many loopholes have been discovered. And it advocates for THS to take several project initiatives on regular-basis for enhancing people's knowledge in line with the suggested recommendations. And it should be taken into consideration, how community will be engaged more for mitigating Health Problems like COVID-19.

REFERENCE

1. Barua, S. (2020). Understanding Coronanomics: The economic implications of the coronavirus (COVID-19) pandemic.

2. Bootsma MCJ, Ferguson NM. The effect of public health measures on the 1918 influenza pandemic in U.S. cities. *Proc Natl Acad Sci* USA. (2007) 104:7588-93. doi: 10.1073/pnas.0611071104

3. IEDCR. Bangladesh Covid-19 Update https://www.iedcr.gov.bd/ (accessed in July 31, 2020)

4. Li Q, Guan X, Wu P, Wang X, Zhou L, Tong Y, et al. Early transmission dynamics in Wuhan, China, of novel coronavirus-infected pneumonia. *NEngl JMed.* (2020) 382:1199-207. doi: 10.1056/NEJMoa2001316

5. Qiu, W., Chu, C. Mao, A. and Wu, J. (2018). The Impacts on Health, Society, and Economy of SARS and H7N9 Outbreaks in China: A Case Comparison Study. Journal of Environmental and Public Health, Volume 2018, Article ID 2710185, 7 pages, https://doi.org/10.1155/2018/2710185.

6. Rahman, M. A., and Islam, M. R. (2020). COVID-19 pandemic: Community engagement could be the best approach for mitigation. Technical Report. July 2020.

7. TMSS Health Sector. https://www.tmsshealth.com/

8. TMSS Working Paper on Health Research. "Report on TMSS Health Care Center (THCC), Bangladesh". December 2019. https://www.tmsshealth.com/rpd-bulletin-2/

9. Worldometers. Covid-19 Pandemic Update. https://www.worldometers.info/coronavirus/ (accessed in June 10, 2020)

Research, Planning & Development Department

The department of Research Planning & Development called in-short as RP&D; has been started its work in 2016 under TMSS Health Sector. The main responsibility of RP&D is to conduct high quality researches in all branches of public health and medical science as well in order to improve the people's livelihood for generating and disseminating new innovation, and knowledge for sustainable development. Formulating plans (Short, Mid and Long-term) for overall development of the Health Sector of TMSS is also the major task of this Department. RP&D has also offered training for professionals and developing high quality human resources for local, regional, national and international purpose.

THE AUTHORS

Md. Matiur Rahman, MBBS, MPH, PhD

Mr. Rahman is working in TMSS since 2003 for health sector in different management positions. Presently he is Deputy Executive Director, responsible mainly for the overall health services and medical educational institutions management. He is also teaching in the department of Public Health under Pundra University of Science & Technology, Bogura, Bangladesh as Associate Professor and Adjunct Faculty of three more Universities and Colleges. He is also in charge of Research, Planning & Development Department under TMSS Health Sector. He has credited a good number of Research and Seminar Papers. He attended in many national and international seminars in home and abroad. Besides, he has visited more than 20 countries in Asia, Europe and America. He is also member of several educational institutions and social organizations. ***Email:*** *dr_matiur@yahoo.com*

Md. Aminur Rahman, PhD

He is known as Development Sociologist having 29 years in Professional career including Teaching, Research and Consultancy in social Development. Dr. Rahman, as a Development Professional has good contribution both Academic and Applied Areas. He has credited two research books and several Articles in national and international Journals. Meanwhile, he contributed as Team Leader nearly 100 research projects on different development areas. Presently, Mr. Rahman is serving as Director of Pundra Institute of Research and Development (PIRD) under Pundra University of Science & Technology, Bangladesh and contributing as the visiting Researcher of South Asian Studies Centre. ***Email:*** *dr.aminur65@gmail.com*

Md. Rahidul Islam

Mr. Islam is working as Junior Researcher of RP&D Department of TMSS Health Sector. Beside this he is serving as Adjunct Faculty of Dept. of Public Health under Pundra University of Science & Technology, Bangladesh. He is doing MPhil degree under Institute of Bangladesh Studies of University of Rajshahi. Before that, he has completed his Bachelor and Masters in social work from the same university at 2013 & 2014 respectively. Mr. Islam has five different publications in National and International Journals on the field of Social Science and Public Health. He has a strong background in Social Science Research Particularly Research Instrument Development, Training of Interviewers, Qualitative and Quantitative Data Analysis, and Report Writing. ***Email:*** *rahidul93.ru@gmail.com*

TMSS Medical College &
Rafatullah Community Hospital
Foundation Office
Thengamara, Rangpur Road,
Bogura-5800, Bangladesh
E-mail: tmsshealth@gmail.com
Web: www.tmsshealth.com

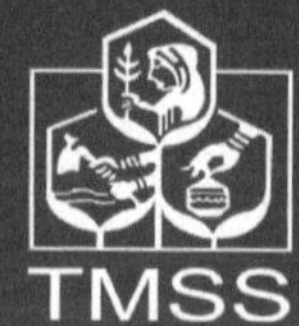

TMSS Head Office
631/5 West Kazipara
Mirpur-10, Dhaka-1216
Telephone: 02-55073586
Fax: 02-55073540
E-mail: tmsseshq@gmail.com
Web: www.tmss-bd.org

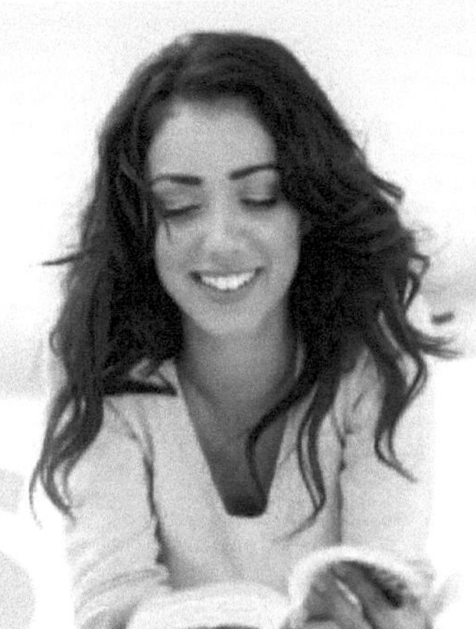

yes I want morebooks!

Buy your books fast and straightforward online - at one of world's fastest growing online book stores! Environmentally sound due to Print-on-Demand technologies.

Buy your books online at
www.morebooks.shop

Kaufen Sie Ihre Bücher schnell und unkompliziert online – auf einer der am schnellsten wachsenden Buchhandelsplattformen weltweit! Dank Print-On-Demand umwelt- und ressourcenschonend produziert.

Bücher schneller online kaufen
www.morebooks.shop

KS OmniScriptum Publishing
Brivibas gatve 197
LV-1039 Riga, Latvia
Telefax: +371 686 204 55

info@omniscriptum.com
www.omniscriptum.com

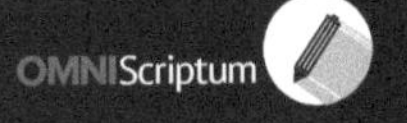

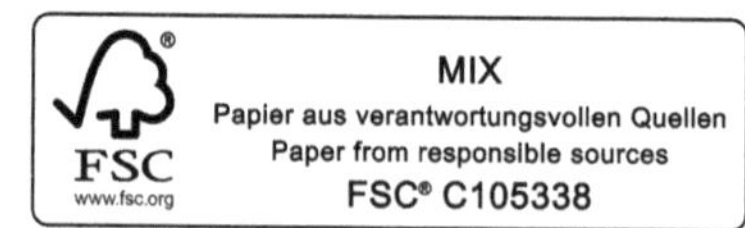

Printed by Books on Demand GmbH, Norderstedt / Germany